M000316154

HEALING HISTORIES

HEALING HISTORIES

Stories from Canada's Indian Hospitals

Laurie Meijer Drees

THE UNIVERSITY OF ALBERTA PRESS

Published by
The University of Alberta Press
Ring House 2
Edmonton, Alberta, Canada T6G 2E1
www.uap.ualberta.ca

Copyright © 2013 Laurie Meijer Drees

Library and Archives Canada Cataloguing in Publication

Meijer Drees, Laurie, 1965–
    Healing histories : stories from Canada's Indian hospitals / Laurie Meijer Drees.

Includes bibliographical references and index.
Issued also in electronic formats.
ISBN 978-0-88864-650-7

    1. Native peoples—Hospitals—Canada—History—20th century. 2. Native peoples—Hospital care—Canada—History—20th century. 3. Tuberculosis—Hospitals—Canada—History—20th century. 4. Tuberculosis—Treatment—Canada—History—20th century. 5. Tuberculosis—Patients—Medical care—Canada—History—20th century. 6. Indian nurses—Canada—History—20th century. 7. Medical care—Canada—History—20th century. 8. Native peoples— Historiography. 9. Oral history—Canada. I. Title.

RA450.4.I53M44 2013   362.1089'97071   C2012-908399-2

"Tuberculosis Thief" by Louise Bernice Halfe, from Bear Bones & Feathers (Regina: Coteau Books, 1994), is reprinted by permission of the publisher.

First edition, first printing, 2013. Printed and bound in Canada by Houghton Boston Printers, Saskatoon, Saskatchewan.
Copyediting and proofreading by Meaghan Craven.
Indexing by Adrian Mather.

All rights reserved. No part of this publication may be produced, stored in a retrieval system, or transmitted in any form or by any means (electronic, mechanical, photocopying, recording, or otherwise) without prior written consent. Contact the University of Alberta Press for further details.

The University of Alberta Press is committed to protecting our natural environment. As part of our efforts, this book is printed on Enviro Paper: it contains 100% post-consumer recycled fibres and is acid- and chlorine-free.

The University of Alberta Press gratefully acknowledges the support received for its publishing program from The Canada Council for the Arts. The University of Alberta Press also gratefully acknowledges the financial support of the Government of Canada through the Canada Book Fund (CBF) and the Government of Alberta through the Alberta Multimedia Development Fund (AMDF) for its publishing activities.

This book has been published with the help of a grant from the Canadian Federation for the Humanities and Social Sciences, through the Awards to Scholarly Publications Program, using funds provided by the Social Sciences and Humanities Research Council of Canada.

Canadä   Canada Council Conseil des Arts   **Government**
          for the Arts du Canada   **of Alberta** ∎

For Marjorie Ward and Marlys Tedin, and

those who experienced Canada's Indian Hospital system

An dah stories you know
dats dah bes treasure of all to leave your family.
Everyting else on dis eart
he gets los or wore out.
But dah stories
dey las forever.

—Maria Campbell
Stories of the Road Allowance People

TUBERCULOSIS THIEF

Playing
On the aspen floors by
Grandma's hearth, memories
drifted of her mama's warmth.

Listening to
the talking box
She heard her mama's voice.

She probed the nylon mesh
poked and shooked the voice box
calling Mama, Mama
Pekīwe, pekīwe.

Hands gripped on the knobs of
the lying box,
she bowed her curly head while
the talking spirits drifted
and took her mama away.

Grandma's hand stroked her
soaking cheeks while
the child of sapling height
thought her mama dead.
The tuberculosis thief
hid in her mama's lungs
and buried her
three years
behind the sanatorium walls.

—Louise Bernice Halfe
Bear Bones & Feathers

CONTENTS

3

4

5

6

OPENING REMARKS

FOR MY FAMILY, HEALING was very important, and we learned and continue to practice valuable methods. In our culture, the plants and medicines have a living essence, or spirit, and it is important to connect prayers and blessings so the mind, body, and living spirit will stay connected. My great-grandparents practiced cleansing methods not only for the mind and the spirit but also for their physical bodies. The cleansing methods use four elements: fire, water, earth, and air. Each of these elements is an important part of the cleansing process.

Belief in the power of these methods was taught to us at a young age and was considered very important. As a result, when we use these cleansing methods, mind, body, and spirit open up to the essence of the ritual. If a person isn't open to the ritual, he or she just goes through the motions and isn't helped—in other words, being skeptical automatically stops the process of healing. The person then will receive no healing. All the rituals strengthen the mind to avoid illness, even contagious illness. The shamans, such as my ancestors, were able to avoid small pox and new diseases upon contact with carriers.

The human mind is empowered when it meets traditional knowledge. That truth was taught to us by Elders through oral history. The mind can be used to destroy the self when not used in a proper disciplined manner. You can be your own enemy and cause an illness; illness can also be caused by others' breath. You can heal yourself or unheal yourself.

The Creator gave us medicines to strengthen us, and these medicines have sustained us through many attacks of different forms, such as pox, measles, leprosy, and mental breakdown. The traditional teachings of my family will carry us through difficult times, and it's wise to share them and care for one another. In that way we receive a blessing and become stronger.

No modern medicines heal—they are temporary and only act on symptoms, and the body doesn't know what to do with them. My uncle never healed at the TB hospital. He became more ill from being confined in the hospital and not seeing his family. The hospital confinement only caused exchange of the tuberculosis germ among patients, spreading it among the confined.

> I'mushstuhw tu Uy shqwaluwun,
> Florence James, Penelakut First Nation
> 2012

PREFACE
"Storywork": Foundations

> The truth about stories is that's all we are.
> —Thomas King
> The Truth About Stories: A Native Narrative

CANADA'S PUBLICLY FUNDED UNIVERSAL health care system repre-
sents an almost sacred hallmark of what we collectively believe defines
Canadian society. Since the early 1960s—as a result of the federal 1957
Hospital Insurance and Diagnostic Services Act and subsequent provincial legislation—access to hospitals, doctors, and associated health
care services are now a part of what most Canadians accept as the
minimum in state-provided social-security programming. Yet, despite
the appearance of universality and equal access, the social history
of medical services in Canada reveals a clear difference in the sub-
stance and delivery of health care to Aboriginal and non-Aboriginal
populations.[1]

The somewhat obscure yet historical fact is that Canada's health care system did not always guarantee universal or equal access to all people living in this nation. Canada's Status Indian, non-Status Indian, Métis, and Inuit peoples' access to Western-style, formalized, institutional health care is different from that of non-Native Canadians, and moreover, each of these Aboriginal groups, representing distinct political–legal entities, has experienced divergent access to those services.[2]

The history of Canada's Indian Health Services (IHS), its workers, and its clients offer many truths. Some of these facts are readily understood while others are more subtle and difficult; all are complex. Foundational to all these stories is the fact that between the 1940s and the 1970s, Canada's federal government offered Aboriginal peoples a *separate* health care service from that available to non-Aboriginal Canadian citizens.

Scholars interpret the history of Aboriginal peoples within the Canadian state in many ways, commonly emphasizing the colonial nature of the relationship between Aboriginal communities and Canada. For the most part, such accounts emphasize the power imbalance between Aboriginal communities and Canada's governments. They also focus on the oppressive policies those governments brought to bear on Aboriginal peoples. Such histories provide invaluable insights into such themes as the control of the state, exploitation of minorities, the nature of resistance movements, and the role of authority in society. These histories focus on interpreting the larger social and political processes within Canadian society and its many constituent communities.

In contrast to those works, this history of Canada's Indian Health Services and its clients draws our attention to something much smaller and closer but equally important: individuals. Here, persons rather than systems and communities are given precedence. Here, we concentrate on the stories told by individuals who experienced the IHS. This work also employs Aboriginal approaches to the sharing of stories. Juxtaposing stories and perspectives, it offers the reader/ listener a chance to grapple with the stories directly as they are passed along from teller to listener, rather than having the accounts interpreted for them through a lens of colonial or critical theory. In fact, the work shared here might be considered postcolonial because it re-orients readers to multiple perspectives as shared through stories rather than a singular history of a series of events. Today, the Truth and Reconciliation Commission of Canada is investigating Indian residential schools as a result of its view that these shared stories of Canada's Aboriginal and non-Aboriginal people are indeed important: "The truth of our common experiences will help set our spirits free and pave the way to reconciliation."[3] I believe that sharing these stories is a form of healing, especially for the storytellers.

Perhaps surprisingly, I began this project as an academic history of nurse training and nursing work in Alaska. In 2000, while working at the University of Alaska–Fairbanks, I searched through archives and interviewed Alaska Native Service nurses and doctors in Fairbanks, Homer, Sitka, and Anchorage. Much as in Alaska, Canada's West and North experienced epidemics of tuberculosis, measles, and other infectious diseases in indigenous communities in the first half of the twentieth century. Among these illnesses, tuberculosis ranked as the worst and most dreaded. When I returned to Canada from Alaska, I was determined to piece together the stories of Canada's IHS, and its impact on families and communities.

Rather than delve into the complex political and administrative history of this federally administered health service, I wanted to focus on the human side of Aboriginal health care based in and on the voices and stories of the people who experienced IHS. My goal was to faithfully present the expressions of Aboriginal people who have rarely, if ever, spoken publicly about their past experiences with Western medicine and Canada's Indian Health Services.

Over several years I continued my research. I found photographs here and there, of tiny babies held by gowned and masked nurses, or of young men and women strapped to stretchers (known as Stryker frames) in hospital corridors, smiling uncertainly into the camera. There were sporadic government records, and I even came across peoples' candid recollections. I travelled around British Columbia,

Alberta, Saskatchewan, and the Yukon, looking for former IHS sites and came across the old nursing stations and hospitals in unexpected places.

Then, in the summer of 2004, I visited Mrs. Kathleen Steinhauer in Edmonton, Alberta. She had worked as a registered nurse in Edmonton's IHS hospital—the Charles Camsell Indian Hospital. She and her husband Gilbert Anderson shared what they remembered about that hospital and all who worked there. Their conversations and warm support gave me the much-needed courage to take on the daunting task of telling a more complete story about IHS. I realized collecting stories from IHS patients and workers was the only way to understand how this institution affected the people it was designed to help. Inspired by Kathleen Steinhauer, I put fresh batteries in my cheap tape recorder and stepped up my work.

Back home on Vancouver Island, I asked around about who might be willing to recall their experience or work with Indian Health Services. Several IHS facilities existed in the coastal British Columbia area, including a large hospital in Nanaimo. Soon enough, people volunteered their precious memories and stories, many of which had remained unrecalled for years. Sometimes opportunities for interviews came as a complete surprise. For example, on my birthday in 2007, my colleague, friend, and Cowichan Tribes Elder, Ray Peter, and his wife Florence Elliott took me on an unexpected trip to visit Ray's cousin, Sainty Morris, who told us about his life in the Nanaimo Indian Hospital. He urged me to share his story with anyone who would listen. Others followed. In all, I collected stories from sixteen individuals to augment other stories I had gleaned from archival recordings.

Still I was faced with my own part in their storytelling, first as a listener, then as a writer. I was bothered by the idea that it was hard for me to fully understand the experiences of the people touched by IHS. This is a challenge facing any person confronted with stories from a place and time removed from their own. Yet, being connected to people who had lived and worked in the Indian Hospital system made me very conscious of the many perspectives this history contained.

In this work I wanted to foreground the stories of the people and not merely record an oral history. Knowing that, I drew a great deal of inspiration from many fine writers and scholars—Aboriginal and non-Aboriginal alike—whose work involved the recreation of narratives, creating a juxtaposition of historic voices. These writers and scholars have grappled with the intricacies and delicacies of sharing life stories and community stories in text.

In particular, a group of Canadian scholars working with Aboriginal narratives have been especially inspiring to me. Julie Cruikshank's Life Lived Like a Story (1987), and her other works, including The Social Life of Stories (1998), reminded me how stories provide frameworks for experiencing the world and that, in doing so, they give people "internal resources to survive" over a lifetime where chance and change are ever-present.[4] Neal McLeod has written eloquently about the significance of narrative in Cree culture, demonstrating how stories, songs, and prayers form the precious collective memory of communities and provide people with food for the soul.[5]

Over the seven years of my story gathering, I learned a great deal, not only from the stories themselves but also about how I could best gather them and present them in a manner that honoured the intent and trust of the storytellers. I also learned hard lessons about the difficulties of documenting stories.

My approach to my work evolved gradually. Most important to my work were valuable lessons passed to me by Maria Campbell, Métis storyteller, writer, and Elder, and Ellen White (Kwulasulwut), Snuneymuxw First Nation Elder, storyteller, and teacher. Maria and Ellen continually emphasized that oral histories are stories and must be shared as such. They reminded me that oral histories are more than answers to structured interview questions. They are instead a part of a person's life—a little bit of personal energy—that must be handled with respect and care, and not simply turned into objects of study. Stories are gifts given, not collected. Both women worked hard to encourage me to approach community stories or personal memories from an Aboriginal perspective—as storytelling moments with all the protocol required of such events.

These two teachers also suggested I write oral histories in a manner consistent with Aboriginal traditions of storytelling. In their respective traditions, and from their perspective, stories are meant to help people, to teach them, and to be shared for the benefit of others. When shared, stories are powerful tools for gaining personal insights about oneself and building relationships between people. Indeed, in her detailed and informative book *Indigenous Storywork* (2008), Stó:lō scholar Jo-ann Archibald (Q'um Q'um Xiiem) calls this approach to Aboriginal stories "storywork."[6] And work it is! Practicing my research as a form of storywork, I gathered the oral histories using techniques quite different from my conventional training as an historian.[7]

First, to exercise respect and reciprocity, I arranged for others to be present during storytelling sessions. Through her patient repetition of the need to work this way, Ellen White taught me that it is better to be with others when sharing stories with an Elder or when stories of personal importance are being told. All my interviews were conducted with people with whom I had some personal connection, or with whom I shared a connection to someone else. My contact with interviewees often came through word-of-mouth recommendations by others—and by invitation.

The presence of more people helps both the listeners and the teller. For the teller, an audience is a welcome presence; for the listeners it is important to have others to discuss or even debrief the story, and ultimately, to help remember it. In my own work, I was often accompanied by Delores Louie (Elder in the Stz'uminus First Nation), by Ray Peter (Elder for Cowichan Tribes), or by colleagues familiar with my project. Only very rarely did I meet alone with a person whose story I was recording. Thanks to my listening partners, I had others to reflect on the stories with, and others with whom to share some of the grief the stories convey.

Sharing stories in a group setting also builds relationships between listeners and tellers and ensures the protocol of proper behaviour is exercised during the telling session. It creates a relational accountability, helping listeners check one another. Because the stories I have been told contain difficult, powerful, and sometimes painful personal insights and experiences, I learned gathering stories could not and should not be rushed. As Florence James, teacher and Elder of the Penelakut First Nation, reminded me, hearing the stories is as much an active effort of "listening" as it is a process of "lessoning."[8] The listener must remember stories are teaching moments. People share their personal experiences for the benefit of others, and the learning process through stories is deliberately slow.

I quickly understood how interview work in this field really only works by invitation, rooted in relationships underwritten by reciprocity and trust. This approach to story gathering has been described by Opaskwayak Cree scholar Shawn Wilson as "simply the building of more relations."[9] By writing down their stories, I engaged in something more than creating an oral history document. The people who shared their stories with me expected me to share them with others; this was the expressed desire of the storytellers. I was also to remain connected to them as long as I worked with their story.

Both my teachers, Ellen White and Maria Campbell, emphasized, each in her own way, the importance of acknowledging and being accountable for my storyteller's role. I had to accept that in the telling, I, too, was a storyteller. It meant not only gathering stories but also sharing my own insights as I passed the stories along to others. It wasn't enough for me to just collect stories, to simply record and edit an oral history. Trusted by the storytellers, my obligation was to insert myself into the life of each story, perhaps to offer my own analysis and to bring an historical context to stories from the people. My teachers told me I was part of a chain along which stories are passed. By extension of these teachings, I challenge readers to bring their own knowledge to the stories. Every person who reads or hears a story becomes part of that story's life and adds meaning to it. In addition, through these stories each listener's life is touched by the events in someone else's. Stories change us; they make us share. Stories are not just a form of pristine evidence, an object outside of us, but are rather a living and lively way of "being together." In fact, stories remind us that we are never alone—as long as we have a story.

The giving, sharing, and transmitting of stories are complex processes in Aboriginal contexts. Obviously traditions and protocols associated with storywork vary between communities, but there does seem to exist a shared understanding that listeners have as much responsibility in the work as tellers. For a listener to fully understand a story he or she must hear it more than once; tellers have to repeat their words often. In turn, listeners must train and discipline themselves to receive the story and the many meanings and lessons it might offer. An open mind hears differently than one that is preoccupied. Tellers and listeners have a special bond with one another in this work. These are concepts my teachers all agreed on.

Overall, through relationship, respect, and reciprocity, my role in my own storywork was to be accountable and contribute to the collective memory of people who had been affected by Indian Health Services. As Canada deals with these stories, like so many others offered to our national Truth and Reconciliation Commission, their true value will become increasingly apparent. How that value will be expressed and acknowledged only future generations will know. Will the stories serve merely as testimonials of Canada's colonizing past? Or as something more grand and inspiring: the strength of communities and cultures? Listeners and readers will decide.

Hearing these stories was but the start of my journey. Once recorded, I began the process of transcription. This meant many hours of sitting at my desk, listening to tapes and typing as fast as I could to keep up with the storytellers. In this process, I wanted to recreate the voice of the teller. Where possible, storytellers helped me confirm their confidence in the final typed version. For those interviews derived from archives, I have noted the source so that readers can find the original interview themselves if needed. In addition, Elders working with me have guided my insights and enriched my understanding and analysis of the historical framework surrounding the stories.

The stories in this book are meant as invitations to consider the world of the teller—a means to examine another view of a complex set of events.[10] They are not, in the first instance, merely autobiographical statements. Instead, they show how people feel about and interpret events, moving listeners/readers beyond the events themselves and into the world of perception and understanding. Each of the narratives presented here offers an opportunity to glimpse a snapshot of a worldview or to accompany another person on a small part in a life's journey.

In this book, several noteworthy themes emerge. With voices of optimism, humour, determination, pride, hope, and strength that echo through the texts, Aboriginal storytellers convey a sense of pride in their ability to overcome the legacy of IHS activity in their own lives. As listeners, we, too, may be healed of our notions of Aboriginal peoples as victims of yet another imposed system as we come to appreciate that their traditional healing practices and notions of health were never really subsumed to Western medicine.[11] First Nations patients and their families continued to understand medicine and well-being in different ways from the established medical professions. Although I can never be wholly certain I successfully fulfilled all the intentions of the people who trusted me with their IHS stories to demonstrate these themes, my wish is that through my storywork I have served well the tellers and their stories and contributed to that healing.

"Food for the soul," as Neal McLeod would say, these stories are more than historical facts; they embody an opportunity—a process—for understanding a period of time that has not been fully described or appreciated, a time that occasionally has slipped into shadow. Through this process, individuals, collective memories, and even a history may be better understood, find more human dimension, and thus heal the pain of real events and injustices that have been obscured and nearly forgotten. We dare not lose sight of this fact, for when a piece of history has been lost, we lose the vital benefit of relationship and respect not only for other peoples' cultural memory but also for our own. In the words of Native American author and storyteller Joseph Bruchac, "Stories have always been at the heart of all our Native cultures...They remind us of the true meaning of all the lives. Our stories remember when people forget."[12]

NANAIMO INDIAN HOSPITAL

A Patient Remembers

Sainty Morris

One morning at Vancouver Island University, after meeting with students and Elders, our Elder-in-Residence, Uncle Ray, asked me what I would be doing the next day. "It's my birthday!" I answered. "Good," he said, "then you can come and pick us up!" He had a plan, but I didn't know it. Both Ray and his wife Flo were ready for me when I went to pick them up on the reserve outside of Duncan, on Vancouver Island. We drove south, took a ferry from Mill Bay to Brentwood Bay, had breakfast in a small roadside café on Flo's insistence, and continued on.

Flo gave me directions to the reserve, from one house to another. Nobody was home. Finally, when Ray knocked on a window, he saw a person inside. After disappearing for a few minutes, he reappeared and waved us in.

We all settled into the front room, where Sainty Morris's grandsons were our hosts. We introduced ourselves, jokes were exchanged, and after a short wait, Sainty came home from work, especially to meet us. Sainty is Ray's cousin, but they thought of each other as brothers.

Sainty's childhood was greatly shaped by the hospital and the formalities of Western medicine. Even his name, "Sainty," came about as a result of an Indian Affairs nurse, who spelled his name incorrectly on his birth certificate. Sainty's aunt tried explaining to the nurse that the baby was to be named "Sandy." The nurse, unable to understand the baby's family, simply entered "Sainty" as the newborn's name.

With Ray and Flo smiling encouragingly, I introduced myself and said that I would like to hear his stories about the Nanaimo Indian Hospital. Sainty leaned forward from his seat on the couch and began. At some points in his story everyone stopped to laugh out loud; at other moments, we all grew quiet. Although the house was cool—the woodstove sat empty—we did not break for tea or any other pleasantries.

Sainty's was the first story I heard that described life inside an Indian hospital from of a patient's point of view. From Sainty's perspective, we learn how the quality of life in the hospital was greatly determined by how close or far a person was from family. Sainty's love of family is a significant theme throughout the account. In vivid detail, he described the hospital routines and treatments, staff attitudes, and educational experiences. His story also illustrates the close connection between the Indian hospitals and the Indian Residential Schools system; the movement of people between the schools and hospitals was ongoing at this time. Significantly, the story ends with the triumph of Indian medicine over hospital treatments.

Sainty told this story virtually without stopping. Only once or twice did Ray add a few details. At the end of the story, we all thanked Sainty for his time. When I offered him an honorarium, he laughed and said he'd gladly tell it all again!

FIRST OFF, MY OLDEST BROTHER was married to a lady from Songhees reserve. This was in 1945. She had very bad tuberculosis, but she wouldn't go to the hospital. That's how she passed it on. They eventually brought her to the Nanaimo Indian Hospital. My brother stayed back at home, and he already had it so bad that he moved in with my parents where all the children still were. He was my oldest brother, and we shared a bed. There was so little room in our house. He was coughing all the time, even in his sleep, and eventually I came down with this sickness, too.

It got so bad after a while that I couldn't get out of bed and walk. One day, when we came home from Yakima, the first thing Mom and Dad did was to bring me to the doctor and then an X-ray. More tests were done and X-rays made, and they told me that I had advanced stages of tuberculosis. They said, "We have to put you in another hospital." They sent me home for a couple of days. Then a nurse came to pick me up and brought me directly to the Nanaimo Indian Hospital.

Being in the hospital was something I was not used to. Right away they started me on needles, and every morning I got a needle in my hip. I was so pockmarked from the needles that they would switch to my other hip and switch back. They had a medication which they called PAS. It was a yellow liquid, bitter tasting, but I got used to it. Then they changed it to another form of PAS in the colour of vanilla. When I think about it now, it makes me wonder. When they put me on the first drug it was as if they were "trying out" things on me, like they were experimenting.

In the hospital the food was good. At the time we were used to our native ice cream [made from berries and fish grease whipped together into a tasty treat] and other food that we were raised on. At that time, my family had little money, and we lived mainly off the land and the beaches. When I was in hospital, I wished I had clams, duck, and all that food from home that I could not have.

The nurses when I first got in there were funny. They were mean and there was one nurse who used the strap on us. I remember a particular time. It was when I first got to the hospital. They had what you called a rest period. It was set for an hour in the morning and an hour in the afternoon. I was new there and could not force myself to sleep so I picked myself up a book, a comic book. As I was lying there reading, I remember how suddenly the book was smashed out of my hand. I got strapped! The nurse took my comic book away and strapped my hand with leather.

On the other hand, there was another nurse who was very friendly. After I got stronger, she would come and take me out, downtown, for a pop and ice cream. The other kids were sure jealous, but she took to me. She did that quite a few times, and I thought she was a very wonderful friend as opposed to the other one. I wasn't the only one that was strapped. She strapped a lot of other children.

I was there off and on for, I can't remember, years, months, days. I was in there for a year and a half when they sent me to Kuper Island Indian Residential School. After being there for a while, I was sent back to the Nanaimo Indian Hospital.

I was allowed to walk around in the hospital since I was BRP. That means bathroom privileged! [laughs] I would walk around the hospital and go visit friends. I got to do this after a year and a half of being in bed. One day the head nurse came to see me, and she told me I was going home. I was so happy! She said, "We are going to measure you for clothing and are ordering your clothes from Vancouver. Then you are going home." A few weeks later, the nurses came and brought me to change into my new clothes. I got a bath and changed clothes, and then I asked if I could visit my friends and relatives. I was allowed to visit, and they said, "We'll find you when the nurse is ready." Miss Fletcher finally showed up, and we got into her car and started heading south, towards where my family lived.

We started going towards Chemainus [a town south of Nanaimo, on the way to Saanich]. I thought we were going to a store there, but when we got to the wharf, she told me to get out. I thought, "What is going on?" She told me, "You are going to Kuper Island Residential School." I told her, "No, they told me I was going home." That's when the nurse told me, "No, I've strict orders not to leave you until you get onto that boat." So I got onto the boat, and they brought me there [to the residential school]. Everyone knew there was a new student coming, and as I was walking up the wharf I saw everyone watching me, whispering, "There he is."

This school was another awful place. They [the hospital staff] didn't tell my parents they were shipping me to Kuper Island! My parents didn't know where I was! My late sister-in-law, Therese, she phoned my parents to ask how I was doing, and that's when it turned out they didn't know where I was. I finally wrote a letter to let them know I was at the school. When I asked the principal why they sent me to Kuper Island, he said that I was here for a rest. Some rest that was. I tell you, I did not know why they did that!

As soon as I got there, they had me scrubbing things on my hands and knees and washing everything by hand. After I finished one place, I had to wax. I had to do every room in that school, both the boy and girl sides. The other kids were in school, and I went to class part of the time. One day they told me to go to the top dormitory and to wash the outside of the building and to be careful not to fall down. There was no rope, no safety, and if there was a streak I would have to go back and clean it. Eventually I got sick again, and I was sent back to the hospital in Nanaimo.

My mom and dad came maybe three or four times during the time I was there. They stayed just for a little while. Money was hard to come by for them—there were no jobs. The only time they had a job was in the summer when they travelled down to the States to work in the berry camps. We always had relatives come over to visit at the hospital, and every Sunday was a visiting day. Family always had to let them know a few days ahead of time if they were going to visit. Some days the hospital officials would let our family visit and some-times not.

Nobody was allowed out of the hospital other than the time when the nurse picked me up. Now and then on a hot summer day, we were allowed out for fresh air, and to suntan on the porch between the girls and guys wards. That hospital was an old army barracks. They demolished it several years back. I can't find any pictures of it. I remember the barracks buildings were all joined together with one central hallway. It was one hallway with lots of wings adjoining it. These wings were lettered up to H. Wings A to G were as follows: A was for older people; B was for teenagers; C housed young babies and toddlers; D is where the young teenage girls were; E was for little older teenagers; F was for young boys; and, finally, G was for older women. The first time I went there, they put me with young boys and when I got shipped back from the Kuper Island Indian Residential School they put me back with older boys.

On Sundays in the hospital, we wrote letters to our pen pals. In those days everyone also had a radio to listen to request shows. We got to write a lot of letters to our pen pals.

There was one teacher I remember from the hospital, but I can't remember her name. She always brought a stack of work, and we were supposed to learn by just reading. No one asked questions. I studied really hard and there were things that I didn't understand. If I asked questions she would explain it really quickly, and then she would be gone again. That went on for the duration of time I was in the hospital. When I went to Kuper Island, they asked me what grade I was in and I told them I thought I was in grade four. So they put me in grade four. As it turned out, I wasn't there for very long, and finally they said they were moving me to grade five.

After they put me in grade five, they suddenly put me off all my duties for a while. The teacher gave me a book and said, "You study that whole book. You have two weeks to study every page." I didn't know what the deal was and I had two weeks to do this. And where do I study? They said, "Wherever you want to study." So I spent my days studying. Finally, after some time, they asked, "Do you know that book by heart?" Then they tested me [on the catechism]. They said, "The reason we are doing this is that we are sending you somewhere and there will be a spelling bee, a contest. We are going to West Saanich." I was so happy! I thought I might be going home, or at least might see my family! They gave me other things to study, but the catechism book was the hardest thing.

The day of the contest we travelled to Saanich, and after competing several rounds I was the only one left standing on our team. The judges said there was a tiebreaker, and I had to compete against a girl to finish the round. I was a visitor so I had to go first. She eventually won, but I did get a cup for that. After the contest, I asked if I could go and visit my mom and dad. They gave me an hour to visit my family. I told my mother, "I can't stay, and if I do you might get in trouble." We went back to school after that.

I ran away from the Nanaimo Indian Hospital. I climbed out the window. We escaped once before I really ran away. That first time my friend and I got as far as the Nanaimo Indian Reserve, but we turned back to the hospital because I was too tired and couldn't make it. We snuck back the same way as we snuck out. No one noticed. After that, my buddy, who was already walking around, came back every day and said, "Let's run away." Finally, one night we did.

The hospital had a watchman who went by every hour on the hour outside the building, with a flashlight. One night, as soon as he went by, we jumped out the window. Out on the street, every time we saw a car coming we hid. We saw the police going to the hospital, and there was a ditch and we jumped down. I lay down and somehow I thought they must have seen us going down there. I told my friend not to move, and the police shone the light on us. Luckily they didn't really see us! We finally made it away from the hospital grounds and went to his mother's house on the Nanaimo reserve. We stayed there a couple of days. My friend asked me what I wanted to do. Did I want to go home? He gave me some clothes, which were too big, but I didn't care as long as I went home. I was actually too scared to go directly home, so I stayed in Duncan with my aunt and uncle for a while.

I was in Duncan for about a month. My aunt and uncle used to always go to the dances and ride around on the horse and buggy. They were the last ones to get around with a horse and buggy, so I used to ride with my uncle Nelson and I used to go visit my other relatives. I was enjoying myself! I used to help my auntie when she was knitting and go to the dances with them. One night we walked over to visit and were sitting there having tea. Suddenly there was a knock on the door! It was my mother and dad! They came running in and grabbed me and took me home.

When I got home, Mom said, "I'll fix you myself." The next morning she went out into the woods and came back with some bark, and stocked up the cooking stove with wood and boiled that bark. She instructed me very carefully. She said, "You are not going to drink anything except what I cooked." I was not allowed to have tea, water, or pop. The drink she made was very bitter, but I acquired a taste for it. I didn't drink it with sugar, just straight. If you taste boiled tea, with a quarter pound of leaves in a little cup, it is very bitter. That's what it tasted like! I kept taking that drink. I started in early January and kept taking it through June.

One day we got enough money to go visit family in the Indian Hospital in Nanaimo. I even went into the hospital with my parents, and as I was walking down the hallway someone grabbed my arm— two head nurses! I said, "Forget it—I'm not coming back!"

These nurses said, "We just want to take your X-ray."

So I said, "Okay, and that is about it. If you put me in here, I'll go out the window again!" They took the X-rays from the front, back, sides of me, and they came back and asked to talk with me in the office. The doctors and nurses started to question me on what I did while I was gone. They asked, "Did you work? Did you take any kind of medication?" They kept asking if I took some type of medication. They really wanted to know how I got this medication. I finally said it was from my mom. Then, of course, they wanted to talk with my mom. I told them that they couldn't because she was back home in Brentwood Bay; they didn't know my mom was visiting in the hospital that day and I didn't want them bothering her!

The good news was that I was all clear—I had no more tuberculosis! My X-rays were clear! I was so happy. When my visiting was all over, I saw my mom and went to where she was and told her what the nurses said. She cried and she said that I was fixed. I still don't know what kind of medication she gave me. Our people have medication for everything. There are some medicines here for women who are expecting—it grows wild right here. There is lots of medication. For example, devil's club is good for diabetes, and if used properly it can cure diabetes—the herb puts it in remission.

INTRODUCTION
"Storytelling": Why We Must Listen

*...I feel the power which the stories still have,
to bring us together, especially when there is loss
and grief.*
          —Leslie Marmon Silko, *Storyteller*

THERE ARE MANY COMPELLING REASONS to tell the stories about
Aboriginal people and Canada's Indian Health Services. There are
just as many as to why we should listen. During the first half of the
twentieth century, the country's western and northern indigenous
communities experienced epidemics of tuberculosis, measles,
and other infectious diseases. Tuberculosis ranked as the worst and
most dreaded. Invading lungs, bone, and other tissue, the tuberculosis
bacterium devastated an individual's health for years at a time. Not
only were people weakened or lost, but so were families and, sometimes, whole communities.

The Canadian government did not always tolerate Aboriginal self-determination in health care, especially when it concerned infectious communicable diseases, such as tuberculosis. As early as 1914, sections of the Indian Act allowed the government to apprehend patients by force if they did not seek medical treatment.[1] Not only could a person be arrested for avoiding treatment, according to these regulations any person subject to the Indian Act was also personally responsible for seeking treatment from a "properly qualified physician."[2] Such regulations did not recognize treatments given by family or community members. In this way, both federal and provincial law applied its weight to Aboriginal communities, forcing the acceptance of Western medicine for the sake of public health.

Whether in the subarctic or on the rainforested northwest coast, non-Aboriginal doctors and nurses, backed by the Canadian government, inserted themselves into the landscape of traditional medicine. Partly driven by compassion, partly inspired by the need to address the "Indian problem" in Canada, the federal government deemed it prudent to centralize Aboriginal health care in the southern regions of the country, effectively segregating delivery of care to indigenous people. In 1953 the Indian Act still supported Indian health regulations that deemed: "If an Indian does not comply with the provincial law either pursuant to directives received from a provincial medical officer or from a medical officer of Indian Health Services or from a doctor designated to act as a medical officer, or even without having received any directive, he remains of course liable to prosecution under section 18 or 21."[3]

Given this kind of governmental legislation and regulation, I began to ask questions about how the broader Canadian society might distinguish between healing bodies and harming living cultures and people through isolation and segregation. There is a very obvious link between the history of Indian Residential Schools in Canada and the Indian Hospital system. This is not to suggest that the effects were the same but simply to indicate that the institutions were connected through both their clients and workers, and through some of their attitudes. Both health and education institutions exercised an authority over the clients and labour force within them. Questions and issues about autonomy and self-determination are central themes in this book. Recognizably similar themes have emerged in the debates and literature about residential schools in Canada.[4]

This book raises the voices of Aboriginal people—the patients, the families, and the communities who were clients or observers of the Indian Health Services system. These people experienced the policies and treatments offered via IHS. They were also the ones who endured the social change brought on by IHS. The stories presented here are powerful and, in many ways, painful, yet they belie a great deal of humour and strength. It was because of the inner power of those who speak about IHS that the stories are shared today.

What caught my attention after listening to, and reading, the many different stories Aboriginal people told about IHS was how optimism and resilience seemed to permeate their accounts. No matter whose voice shared an insight into the IHS and its workings, somehow a sense of determination and hope shone through. Just as the administrators, doctors, and nurses of IHS believed in their manifest destiny to apply Western medicine in Aboriginal communities, so, too, Aboriginal people tell stories that resonate with a pride in their ability to prevail in the face of impacts Indian Health Services had on their own lives.

Although it might appear that Aboriginal peoples were passive clients of this system, stories, photographs, and disparate records show that many were part of the IHS labour force. In fact, the lines between patient and worker within IHS were sometimes blurred when former patients became employees. In these stories, I found themes of pain, loss, and crisis but also of resilience, achievement, humour, and hope—strengths of the past that can speak to present generations through shared stories.

My storywork also revealed that, although IHS strove to extend modern medical practice and technology to many of the communities under its jurisdiction, Aboriginal peoples' own medical knowledge and practices persisted, often quietly and privately, and sometimes as open resistance to the Western medical system.[5] In fact, many indigenous practices related to health and wellness simultaneously occupied the same space as the treatments offered within the Indian Hospital system of IHS. This reality was not always understood or appreciated by non-Aboriginal IHS employees. From the perspective of many Aboriginal peoples, Indian Health Services offered a service that could be utilized as a commodity—that is, accessed at the will of the patient. If individuals believed that the medical treatment did not suit them, they would or could seek assistance within their own traditions, communities, and families. Sometimes this was done overtly, sometimes covertly. Countless oral histories of Aboriginal peoples' encounters with Western medicine attest to this level of self-determination.

Consistent with the theme of cultural autonomy and traditional health care, another theme I came to appreciate over and over again was the persistence of indigenous "medicines" and their parallel use with Western medicine. Through the stories, I learned that local or traditional healing practices and notions of health were never totally subsumed to Western medicine, and that First Nations patients and their families continued to understand medicine and well-being in different ways from Western medical professions. Quite simply, Aboriginal medicine was never entirely undervalued or discarded; Western medicine came alongside and sometimes dominated the health care of Aboriginal people, but it failed in its presumptive role of extinguishing the authority and efficacy of indigenous concepts of medicine and "health."

Understanding the disease of tuberculosis and how it plagued Western society before its cure emerged is key to setting the stage for the reactive nature of the federal government's plan to isolate and control the epidemic in Canadian society and avoid the transfer of diseases to non-Aboriginal citizens. I cover this in Chapter 1. In Chapter 2 I outline some of the underlying reasons for the creation of Indian Health Services, which, principally, was a response to the epidemics such as smallpox, measles, influenza, and especially tuberculosis that ravaged Aboriginal populations. Indian Health Services was a system that grew out of an older health care structure originally controlled by the Department of Indian Affairs. It was an extensive system, with large and small hospitals, health centres, nursing outposts, and numerous staff.

Following that, in Chapter 3, I describe the institutions of IHS: primarily the hospitals, how they looked and how they worked. Because IHS was a complex patchwork of people, buildings, and jurisdictional questions and issues, it is almost impossible to capture it in a simple description. Yet, it is important to imagine the physical system in which Aboriginal and non-Aboriginal people related to one another.

In Chapter 4, the experiences of Aboriginal families, communities, and individuals are explored. How were families and communities touched by the Indian hospitals? What were the daily experiences of patients? No one was left unaffected by the impact of Indian Health Services and all its related institutions. Even healthy people in Aboriginal communities were often connected to the health care system through an ill relative.

Chapter 5 offers readers the chance to consider indigenous medicines and their continued role both inside and outside formal health care institutions. In Coast Salish territory, cultural teachings related to health and wellness played a significant role in the IHS system, even though their workings were invisible to those unfamiliar with them. Perhaps in other parts of Canada, ancient cultural understandings of illness, how to relieve it, and ideas of wellness were as significant as on the northwest coast in the region of the Nanaimo Indian Hospital. Only more research in the form of oral history will reveal additional truths.

Finally, in Chapter 6 I investigate the place of Aboriginal people as workers within the Indian Health Services system. Although the Indian Hospital system is commonly portrayed as one of non-Aboriginal workers dealing with Aboriginal patients, in fact many workers within the system were Aboriginal. What types of work did they do? How were they trained and hired? Readers who are interested in this area are also directed to the book, *Twice as Good: A History of Aboriginal*

Nurses, recently published by the Aboriginal Nurses Association of Canada (2007), which discusses important and unsung histories of their membership.

Rather than delve into a complex political and administrative history of health and health care here, I want to offer a social history of Aboriginal health care in Canada. And perhaps more important, any political and administrative history, or theoretical comments, are meant only as a—albeit perhaps essential—backdrop to the stories offered by Aboriginal peoples. In *Healing Histories: Stories from Canada's Indian Hospitals,* stories, photographs, and documents merge to bring a new dimension to the ways Aboriginal people—both individuals and communities—were affected by formal health care after the Second World War. Most of my analysis deals specifically with First Nations in northwestern Canada because this is where IHS concentrated the majority of its facilities, regular services, and activities. I illustrate how policies devised by the federal government for Aboriginal health were complex and often contradictory in the decades after the Second World War. Those political visions were often more hopeful than helpful—and, by far, more idealistic than realistic.

The memories of those who worked in or encountered that system provide a convergent view of "what it was." Illustrating this history through the stories and comments of those who were subjected to IHS, this book features the voices of patients, administrators, staff, and interested politicians. They were the ones who felt the actual— rather than the theoretical—workings of that system.

IHS shaped lives and was, in turn, shaped by them. The legacy of IHS is now expressed in efforts made by Aboriginal people to restructure their publicly funded health care in a manner that better reflects their own cultural understandings of what constitutes "health" and "care." Their efforts continue on many fronts—*Healing Histories: Stories from Canada's Indian Hospitals* is one of them. Through this book, they share their stories and contextualize them within a social history of IHS in order to contribute to a reawakened collective memory.

"COLD NEEDLES"[1]

Laura Cranmer

OPENING: A Letter to Dr. Needles

Dear Dr. Needles,

You're probably wondering how we turned out. I'm not sure if you
know this or not, but despite your best efforts, the experiment was
spectacular failure. Well in my case anyway.

I'm sixty this year and your cancer-inducing vial must have been
a dud because I'm still alive, still kicking and still carrying on with
the traditional ways of my people. But for a lot of my friends and relatives, they never made it—thanks to you and all the people involved
with your experiment.

How does it feel to achieve your dreams and professional goals?
Did you ever publish the results of your experiments? How would it
sound to go around bragging about how you sped up the assimilation process by injecting amnesia inducing substances into whole
populations of Indian people?

Here we are trapped in our little beds in our little rows HOG
TIED—TONGUE TIED—WITH OUR BRAINS FRIED tears cuz all
you guys could think of was your fricken mandate and your fricken
theories so righteous were you in your conviction about the projected
results of the experiment.

Signed,
Your patient

SCENE: Dr. Needles at the First Project Forget Meeting— a room full of physicians

Dr. Needles: The government, more specifically the Department of
National Defence and Indian Affairs have made their vast store of
resources available to us (us being select members of the medical
community) to assist in the assimilationist efforts for the Indian
populations of Canada. Despite the best efforts of the missionaries,
churches and Indian agents, the change process is very slow. So
government authorities are now placing their faith more in science
than religion. It is our sacred duty to help these people progress and
assume their proper place in society.

We have all heard how many of the native children are dying
from TB in the residential schools and we all know how the conditions of the schools help to spread the disease. The Indian hospitals
provide the perfect cover for Project Forget because they are perfect
labs, really. We have a much more tightly controlled environment to
monitor the experiments and a much more tightly controlled patient
population. This project is secret of course, and only those in this
room will be privy to what is really going on.

The Indian communities, the missionaries and the Indian agents
have no knowledge whatsoever about our experiment and for this
reason I expect that everyone here will sign an oath of silence for the
rest of your lives. The Indian agents will know about our efforts on a
need to know basis only. We will be using data gathered from other
totalitarian regimes to advance the use of amnesia drugs, truth serums,

cancer-causing agents and other drugs that we feel will help either phase these people out, or phase their customs out, at the very least.

Dr. Forget: Yes, I concur with Dr. Needles. Secrecy is of the utmost importance. We need to remember that what we do here is for the greater good of all Canadian society. Our work will continue to impact on many more generations of Indian people yet to come. Dr. Needles, how will we explain our increased correspondence to the Indian agents and principals of the residential schools?

Dr. Needles: Yes, there are several things to keep in mind. We need to cast our language in as ambiguous terms as possible, something like your high-school English teacher or your Department of National Defence bureaucrat—take your pick.

Dr. Forget: Okay. I pick the DND bureaucrat over the English teacher any day—cuz he can cover my ass while covering his own.

Dr. Needles: We also need to generate public fear about the necessity of keeping a tight control on TB patients who are fighting to go home—we must monitor all in-coming and out-going mail at the hospitals so as not to have word get out of the system about how these patients might be used for experiments.

We must impress upon the Indian agents, the residential school principals and secretaries that the TB situation has spun out of control and we, as government employees, are charged with the highest responsibility of getting things under control. No matter how long it takes. Even though newly touted antibiotics are proving very effective against the TB bacterium, there must be other medical reasons for detaining the patients much longer than they would reasonably expect to stay with the new treatment.

As well, we need to establish a protocol for moving patients between the residential schools and the hospitals. The local RCMP detachments will be notified that they should be vigilant in guarding against possible runaways from either institutions.

Dr. Forget: And how are we to explain to the unsuspecting nurses about the vials of experimental serums for the patients?

Dr. Needles: By keeping a parallel set of records, one for the regular patients who are not part of the experimental program and one for the patients who are part of Project Forget, as overseen by Nurse Colde. We can maintain the strictest security for Project Forget.

SCENE: Faith, a Kwakwaka'wakw nurse in the Indian hospital—sitting on a metal hospital chair.

Faith: One of my white friends says that if he was Indian he wouldn't let anyone with a needle within ten feet of him because he's convinced that the proliferation of Indian hospitals is really a ruse, a façade, a way to recruit patients for covert lab experiments. Of course he doesn't have any evidence to support these outlandish claims.

Speaking of outlandish, as one of the first Indian nursing students, I was seen as outlandish, an anomaly, an aberration. I was treated like a kind of pet seal, "hear her bark! See her clap her hands!" They think I'm incapable of abstract thought and attribute my success to rote memory and dumb luck. But if I let those things get in my way I wouldn't be working here today. The discrimination and loneliness, at times, worked against my dream of graduating. My grandparents' support was my sole anchor.

When I was going through my change as a young woman, they held a small ceremony and charged me with the responsibility of maintaining the healing tradition handed down to us by our ancestors. I remember the cradle songs my grandfather used to sing to me as a little one. He made me laugh with his funny faces and I remember feeling loved and safe and most of all I remember his tenderness. He used to sing all the time.

[The 'Namgis cradle song is played at a low volume—then the character picks up the tune where the tape leaves off—she sings a stanza in Kwak'wala.]

I used to sing in my little girl voice, mimicking his words and face and then it was his turn to laugh. Then I was sent away to a very large building with many many other children who were dressed very oddly and looked at me with pity when I first arrived. There were bells ringing all the time and lines of kids for almost everything you needed to do—from getting food to going to the bathroom to getting medicine to getting Saturday canteen.

After the supervisor cut my hair she made me get into something that I'd never seen before, a kind of indoor waterfall that hit your body like cold needles that stung me all over. All I could do was shiver and look up to see this noisy cold spray hitting my face. So to comfort myself I started to sing the song my grandfather sang and all of a sudden the supervisor pulled me out of the shower by my hair and yelled at me not sing in my language.

And then I caught TB in the school so I was sent, at first to what they called the preventorium or sanatorium, which was blocked off from the rest of the school. They thought with rest I might get better. But I got worse so that I could hardly make sense when I spoke and I couldn't really walk. So I was sent from there to the Indian hospital all the way down Vancouver Island in Nanaimo.

I don't recall very much of my stay there and what I do recall is accompanied by flashes like lightning or an old-fashioned camera with one of those giant flash pans that blinds you every time it goes off.

SCENE: Hospital—Patient Dorothy is in bed.

[Bright white hospital walls with old-fashioned white iron beds—sounds of kids crying—sounds of chaos—sounds of metal pans clanking. A nurse's voice comes over the PA system, "Calling a doctor to Ward B—will Dr. Needles return to Ward B—I repeat will Dr. Needles please return to Ward B!!"]

Dorothy: Nurse can I have some water? My throat is really dry. Please, nurse?

Nurse: [Rushing by with a tray] Yes, yes, I'll be right there Dorothy!

Dorothy: Help. I'm trapped here in this little box and I'll be trapped here for the rest of my life! You think I'm joking, don't you? Well maybe I am and maybe I'm not. But from what I hear—patients like me don't usually walk out of the hospital. We're carried out. They say I'm not growing the way I should be growing. I overheard the nurses whispering about me. They forget my other parts are working...like my ears! And my brain works perfectly well, almost too well! Nurse Wellington told the new nurse she had to watch out for me and she meant it in a mean way. What's to watch out for? I didn't do anything to her! But anyway Wellington whispered that [Dorothy mocks whispering], "she has *osteogenesis imperfecta*," and the other nurse just nods like she knows. Well I don't know. *Osteo. Osteo.*

SCENE: **An old radio on a hospital bedside table.**

[The old radio is playing and crackles out a song.]

Song title: "Isolation:"
    Not supposed to swear,
    Sneak or tear around down the hallways
    Those yawning terrifying hallways
    Not supposed to run around like other kids do
    Why, what'll happen to you?
    You'll get transferred to Isolation
    Isolation that damned Isolation Room
    Where they'll teach you a lesson or two

1

TUBERCULOSIS

 ～～～～～～～～～～～～～～～～～～～～～～～～～～～～

Regardless of the cause or causes, the problem still remains of how to get the Indians and Eskimos to accept the truths of modern hygiene.
—*Ethel Martens, Advisor, Medical Services, 1966*[1]

WEIGHT LOSS AND FEVER. Wracking coughs. Blood in the sputum. Large, rubbery, swollen glands in the neck. Extreme fatigue. These symptoms all characterize tuberculosis or TB—a devastating global disease with an array of debilitating effects and, until the latter part of the last century, a high mortality rate.[2] Although people commonly associate the disease with a lung infection, tuberculosis can also attack the bones, including the spine, as well as a person's internal organs and glands.

It is important to understand something of the epidemiology and history of this disease in order to fully understand why it became a focal point of health care for Aboriginal people in Canada and how reactive government policies concerning TB were a major factor leading to a segregated health care system for First Nations.

For millennia, tuberculosis was a life-threatening disease for which no cures existed. TB's co-evolution with human societies throughout the world is ancient. Archaeological evidence suggests TB existed in Ancient Egypt, Asia, Greece, and Europe; it has existed in North and South American Aboriginal populations for at least three hundred years. TB epidemics have repeatedly swept through human communities regardless of social, cultural, or economic environments. In Europe the last major TB epidemic appears to have peaked in the eighteenth century; a similar epidemic moved through North America the late 1800s and early 1900s, when it is estimated at least 70 per cent of the population was infected with the bacterium. Although not everyone became sick with the disease, a large majority of the population were carriers of TB.

Currently researchers estimate that a third of the world's population is infected with the latent form of TB.[3] The World Health Organization acknowledges that though the proportion of active cases is not increasing, world population growth means the disease—especially in the developing world—is still a significant factor in mortality rates.[4]

Until the 1960s our knowledge about TB, its symptoms, and its spread was limited because of the lack of consistent statistics and public health records related to the disease. Even today the impact of tuberculosis on communities past and present is still not well understood because the disease can be either latent or develop slowly in individuals; people carry the disease for their entire lifetime. An active TB infection is a "slow" disease, one that gives little warning of its presence in the early stages.

Tuberculosis is caused by a tiny bacterium with the Latin name *Mycobacterium tuberculosis* and can affect people of any age or background. Although it was formerly believed tuberculosis bacteria survived on surfaces in an unclean environment, modern research demonstrates that air quality and quantity is a far greater factor in the spread of this disease. TB cannot survive in adequately ventilated environments. In a well-aired house or room, TB droplets suspended in the air are dispersed and have less chance of infecting a new host. Tuberculosis is spread almost exclusively person-to-person through the air or by physical contact. Tiny moisture droplets in the air carry the bacteria, and once those droplets are inhaled by an uninfected individual they are drawn deep into the lungs, where they cause a new infection.

Not all infected people become sick, however. In a healthy person, once these bacteria enter a new host's lungs, the immune system usually manages to engulf and contain the bacteria. The TB bacteria then remain dormant in the body for decades in small walled-off "tubercules." This type of latent tuberculosis infection may never develop into illness; on the other hand it can also re-awaken years later and develop into an active "secondary" tuberculosis infection. In a person with a weaker immune system, the initial bacterial infection might infect and severely damage any part of the body, from lungs and lung tissue, to bones, the spine, glands, and organs.

Outside factors also play a role in how tuberculosis affects a person. Stress, malnutrition, and other illnesses play a large role in exacerbating the disease. Age is also a factor. Various forms of TB appear among people of certain ages—adults are more likely to contract pulmonary (lung) TB, while children are particularly susceptible to extrapulmonary (bone, lung, organ) TB.[5] Pulmonary and extrapulmonary TB may co-exist in a single patient.

Only in the twentieth century did medical research in Europe and the United States establish the origins of this illness and explain its nature. By the middle of the 1900s, the development of drug treatments finally offered hope to anyone who might contract this dreaded illness.

Early treatments of TB were just that: treatments, not cures. Before the discovery of bacteria as the cause of TB, doctors identified the disease as "consumption"—a disease they believed was caused by unclean urban habitats. Considered a disease of the slums and of poor debauched people, conventional wisdom of the day held that TB could seep into a person through environments that were too dark, too damp, dirty, or otherwise considered "immoral." As a result, in the mid-nineteenth century, when TB was still very common in Europe and North America, traditional treatment sought to reverse the conditions responsible for it by advocating that TB patients seek abundant sun, fresh air, and outdoor environments considered physically and morally "clean."

Principally, upper-middle-class TB patients sought to get away from the dirty air of cities to seek comfort in the fresh country air, preferably in a location with plenty of sunlight and a relaxing lifestyle.[6] Euro-American patients travelled as far away as Egypt or as close as the French Riviera or the Swiss Alps, seeking healthy places to recover from TB. Other remedies included spending time at high altitude, or places considered to have unique air qualities.[7] Some people considered rich foods and exercise as viable in treating the disease.

Even after 1882 when German scientist Robert Koch discovered the tuberculosis bacterium that caused TB, treatments for the disease changed little. For the most part, infected individuals were isolated from healthy people and encouraged to rest their lungs. In fact, in the late nineteenth century Europe, the primary treatment for TB became a "rest" cure. Patients would enter a sanatorium—a large rest home where fresh air, good food, and clean surroundings in the country offered hope of a cure. A typical rest cure lasted two years, sometimes longer. Until the discovery of antibiotics in the twentieth century, sanatorium treatment was considered the only option for Europeans and North Americans who discovered they were infected and sick.

By the 1890s and through to the 1950s, surgery in hospitals and sanatoria offered new hope to patients. Doctors devised methods for collapsing patients' lungs, hoping this would rest the infected tissue and lead to healing. A variety of lung- and chest-related procedures and operations emerged, including pneumonectomy—removal of part of a lung—thoracoplasty—removal of ribs—pneumothorax—injecting air into the chest to collapse the lung—and plombage and oleothorax procedures, which involved the injection of nitrogen,

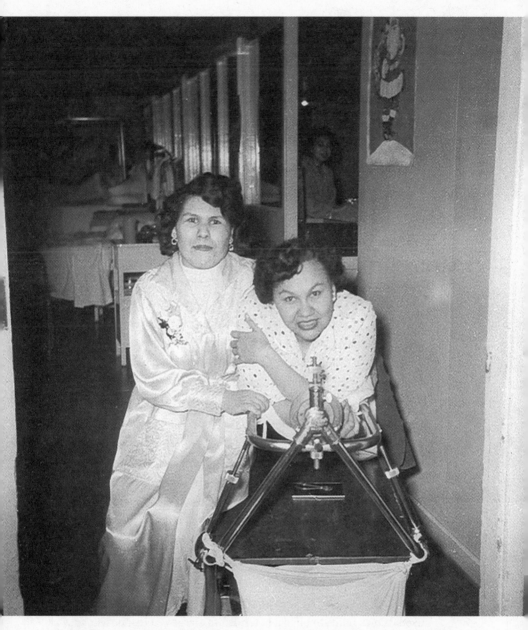

Two friends smile at the camera from their ward hallway at the Charles Camsell Indian Hospital, Edmonton, 1950s. A common treatment for patients with bone tuberculosis was to immobilize them on a Stryker frame (pictured here) in order to limit their movement and protect fragile bones, especially the spine. [PAA 91.383.85]

paraffin wax, rubber sheeting, or mineral or olive oil into the chest cavity to prevent a lung from re-inflating. Other body parts infected with TB were also "rested"—bone TB patients were often placed in casts or splints to stabilize and rest their spines or other long bones, while others were horizontally immobilized in half-body casts or on stretchers ensuring they didn't strain their skeletal system.[8]

In Canada the medical assault on TB looked much like it did in Europe and the United States in the early to mid-twentieth century. In this initial phase, people fought to change the environment in which TB thrived. Prior to the Second World War and the creation of Canada's nationalized health care system, provincial and national organizations, including charities, women's organizations, Church groups, and medical associations, all cooperated to fight TB. Together, they sought to clean up slums, collect money to build sanatoria, improve sanitation in poor neighbourhoods, and even pass anti-spitting laws.[9] In Montreal, for example, the board of trade and the local council of women fought for anti-TB laws, while the Sisters of Providence in Quebec provided nurses to fight the disease.[10]

The end of the nineteenth century ushered in a dramatic therapeutic shift in the treatment of TB with the "Sanatorium Era." In 1896 the National Sanitorium Association built the first Canadian sanatorium, Muskoka Cottage, in Gravenhurst, Ontario. In Ontario others followed in quick succession, and the movement spread across Canada to encompass sixty-one sanatoria by 1938.[11] In the West, for example, the Rocky Mountain Sanatorium in Frank, Alberta, opened during the First World War and operated until the Central Alberta Sanatorium at Keith was opened in 1920. That same year in Calgary, Alberta, the new Central Alberta Sanatorium was built for the ongoing care of tubercular veterans of the First World War.[12] Close to that city, the Blackfoot Indian band—now known as the Siksika First Nation— used its own funds to build a new hospital, largely in response to deal with tuberculosis.[13] In 1916 the sanatorium at The Pas, Manitoba, opened its doors to the public, followed by Saskatchewan's Fort Qu'Appelle Sanatorium in October 1917.

Despite these "rest" and surgical treatments, North American TB infection and death rates continued to be high until the Second World War. In the United States in the 1920s, TB caused 6 per cent of all deaths, or a mortality rate of 97 per 100,000.[14] In fact, TB's impact on U.S. society was greater than polio, although polio gained a great deal more attention.[15] In Canada infection rates also ran high. For example, in Saskatchewan in 1921 44 per cent of children were infected with TB by the age of six. By the age of eighteen, 76 per cent of these children were infected. [16] In Canada in 1926, the mortality rate for TB was 84 per 100,000; in 1939 that rate had dropped to 54 per 100,000 but infection rates remained relatively high, at 88 per 100,000.[17]

In 1943 a huge breakthrough occurred in TB treatment. At Rutgers University, researcher and scientist Selman Waksman developed an antibiotic called streptomycin from the *Streptomyces griseus* bacteria, and soon after doctors at the Mayo Clinic pioneered TB treatment with this new drug. Although physicians had been using penicillin for a few years, it had proved useless in any fight with TB, but the new streptomycin antibiotic represented a major breakthrough in chemotherapy against the disease. Streptomycin had its drawbacks: it had to be administered intramuscularly or intravenously by a nurse or doctor, and the TB bacteria quickly began to develop a resistance to it. The large and painful needles used to inject streptomycin in patients are something few of those who felt them will ever forget.

Once the role of bacteria in TB infection became clear, Canadian efforts shifted more toward in-patient medical treatments and procedures for patients with TB. Now, the aim was to cure, not merely control, the disease. In the 1930s and 1940s X-ray teams spread out across Canada seeking out infected people in mass surveys. Although the Second World War challenged all available resources, from medical personnel to medical equipment and supplies, in the 1940s more sanatoria were built, medical personnel displaced by the war in Europe were employed, and even the Department of Veteran Affairs set up temporary beds and clinics in addition to its Veteran Affairs' hospitals to meet the high demand for its military patients arriving home in the 1940s.

Vaccination programs were launched in Canada: after 1946 every province participated in TB vaccination. From the late 1930s through the 1950s, at least one-third of patients with pulmonary (lung) TB were subject to new surgeries to induce lung collapse, including more thoracoplasty, pneumothorax, and plombage procedures. Streptomycin was distributed widely across Canada after 1948.[18]

Then, in 1949, streptomycin was combined with another new antibiotic known as PAS (para-aminosalicylic acid). This drug was available in pill form, and although terrible tasting and administered in huge doses (twenty-four large blue pills a day), it gave new hope to doctors and patients. Used together, the two drugs proved to be a "cure" for TB. By 1953 drug companies developed isoniazid (INH), another drug that could be combined with streptomycin or PAS. INH was easier for patients to take and proved very effective in slowing TB bacteria growth and killing the bacteria entirely.[19]

After 1950, in addition to straight bed rest, drug treatments with INH or PAS became standard tuberculosis treatments. INH and PAS were taken orally, but PAS was more of a problem for patients because doctors and nurses knew this drug was not easy to handle by patients at home because of the size and number of tablets one needed to take per day. Some patients had a unique form of rebellion. An Alaskan newspaper carried the following account of how patients dealt with their pills.

Dr. Robert Fraser, a former public health service doctor who also served as Alaska's TB control officer, said he remembered going to the children's orthopaedic section and looking out the windows at a lower section of the hospital. "The roof was stained [blue] with PAS," he said. "Th[e] kids didn't like it. It was a lot of pills, it caused an upset stomach, and if you chewed it up it tasted terrible."[20]

Many patients, Aboriginal and non-Aboriginal alike, recalled the streptomycin injections as painful, and the pills as horrible, and not all of them understood the significance of the medications.

The use of these powerful drugs marked the biggest change in TB treatment for two main reasons. First, the drugs were effective in slowing the disease and eliminating the bacteria. Second, PAS and isoniazid were portable and could be used at home rather than having to be administered in a hospital. By the mid-1950s, outpatients typically received drug treatments rather than hospital or surgical treatment, and their healing was faster and more dramatic than ever before. In fact, the new drugs were so effective that by 1960, sanatoria had practically vanished from the landscape of TB treatments.[21]

The TB epidemic in Canadian society in the 1930s, 40s, and 50s drastically affected Aboriginal communities across the country. In the words of an X-ray technician who brought one of the first X-ray teams to Aboriginal communities in northern Manitoba: "It was well known that Native Indian people were very susceptible to tuberculosis. But prior to 1948 little had been done to look for and treat this disease among these people in the remote areas."[22]

In fact, infection rates for TB in Canada's registered Indian population were ten times the national average in 1944. Their infection rates remained significantly higher than the national population into the 1960s.[23] For many Indian people, the Indian Residential Schools system served as their point of infection. Other conditions, such as poverty and crowded living conditions on reserves and in remote communities further supported the spread of TB. These high infection rates drew a great deal of federal government attention and became an important reason for the extension and intervention of formal Western medicine to Aboriginal communities across Canada.

Superficially, the treatment of Aboriginal patients appeared identical to that of other Canadians—though in the 1930s they were rarely offered sanatorium care.[24] Eventually, registered Indian and Inuit patients were taken into sanatoria and hospitals run by government or churches. There, treatment included rest regimes, surgeries, and drugs much like those offered to non-Aboriginal patients.

Still, the health care offered to Aboriginal people was different than that for non-Native people. First, virtually no long-term TB treatment was made available in the territories where indigenous patients themselves lived. Aboriginal patients generally travelled great distances from home to get medical help. Second, to further complicate matters, after 1945, and as wards of the state, Indian and

Inuit patients received treatment in the separate segregated Indian health system, rather than in public provincial facilities. Significantly, this new Western formal health care mostly ignored the cultural and language barriers existing between Aboriginal and non-Aboriginal peoples. At times, some patients believed that the medications were experimental and were fearful of their treatments; others were more accepting.

Third, perhaps most important, it appears the health care extended to Aboriginal peoples was not subject to the same standards of care or consent. In fact, at times Canada's Aboriginal population was used as a "test" population for new drugs or TB interventions. For example, in 1933, noted anti-TB crusader Dr. R.G. Ferguson, director of the Fort Qu'Appelle Sanatorium in southern Saskatchewan, began the first vaccination trials of the BCG (Bacillus Calmette-Guérin) vaccine in Canada. His trial group: infants born within the Qu'Appelle Indian Health Unit. By 1938 his results from his twelve-year trial on this Native population demonstrated the effectiveness of the vaccine, after which it was used on Canada's non-Native population.[25] Even today, those who recall their TB treatments from the 1950s and 1960s often still express a belief that they were being experimented on by the doctors and nurses.

How Canada's Aboriginal people experienced tuberculosis and the formal Western medical care for TB is complex. As patients in special "Indian" hospitals, away from family and community, thrown together with patients speaking many different languages and not English or French, they had little or no voice in their care. Despite their isolation, however, many experienced a remission of their TB and now share their individual memories. In this way they are shaping an important part our collective memory: the history of tuberculosis and Indian health care in Canada.

2

INDIAN HEALTH SERVICES
An Evolving System

The government does not want to be paternalistic, to spoon-feed either group.
It aims rather at putting the Indians and Eskimos in a position to maintain
themselves.
> —Hon. Paul Martin, Radio Broadcast, Ottawa, 1947[1]

The Indian hospitals are good hospitals. There is no over-extravagance. They are
not comparable in some respects with the material set-up of corresponding institutions, although service is good and is one that this country can be proud of, in
keeping with its duty.
> —Hon. Paul Martin, House of Commons Radio Broadcast,
> Ottawa, 1952[2]

After I graduated with my RN designation, I went to work in the Indian hospital
in Edmonton. That was the Camsell, and I started on the pediatric ward. The conditions there were pretty bad. The babies were all dried with the same towel! I
had to petition hard to get separate towels and towel racks for each baby patient.
Some things were just improper.
> —Kathleen Steinhauer, First Nations RN, Edmonton,
> August 25, 2004[3]

INDIGENOUS PERSPECTIVES on health and health care as delivered by Canada's former Indian Hospital system form a significant and little discussed part of Canada's medical history. Yet, to understand these perspectives, the history of federal involvement in Aboriginal health and health care must be sketched to provide a context for the experiences of Aboriginal peoples. The brief history provided here describes governmental efforts, initially under the auspices of the Department of Indian Affairs, to patch together Church- and state-run medical services (1890–1945), followed by the emergence of Indian Health Services (1945–62), the merger of the IHS with other federal health programs into the Medical Services branch, and ultimately the progressive dismantling of the system in the 1970s, when responsibility for health services was finally devolved from government to First Nations bands themselves. A significant trend in the changing government services over time was the shift from a paternalistic model of health care delivery to one that sought to implement abiding cultural change in its Aboriginal clients.

Department of Indian Affairs, 1890–1945

Between the 1890s and 1930, the Department of Indian Affairs controlled initiatives related to the health and health care for Canada's Indian and, later, Inuit peoples. During this period, the department supported both the growth of a medical service within the government and the existence of Church-run hospitals and care facilities. The gradual expansion of formal, Western-style medical services to Aboriginal people came in response to two main factors: public pressure and the widely held opinion that diseases like tuberculosis might spread from the Native to the non-Native community. As a result, expenditures for Indian health grew in the early twentieth century from several thousand dollars annually to $330,625 by 1930 for the western territories alone.[4]

The number of medical personnel also grew during those early years. For example, in 1904 a new medical superintendent was appointed for Indian health, and medical personnel in the federal employ rose from twenty-six medical officers in 1904 to ninety-seven by 1927.[5] From 1936 to 1945, the Indian Affairs branch, under the Minister of Mines and Resources, continued delivering medical care to Indian peoples—and, sporadically, to Métis and Inuit people—through a patchwork of federally operated Indian hospitals and mission hospitals, augmented by a field army of medical officers and nurses.

Until 1945 the piecemeal but growing services to Aboriginal peoples operated as a marriage of Church and state. Aboriginal populations in the southern provinces were served primarily by federal Indian hospitals. Northern locations, like the Northwest Territories, were served entirely by mission hospitals, which were partially, although inconsistently, funded through Indian Affairs.

Indian Health Services 1945: New Directions

In 1945 the freshly constituted federal Department of National Health and Welfare launched a new health care bureaucracy called Indian Health Services. In doing so, it consolidated and reorganized health services for Canada's indigenous communities.[6] After the war, both the newly formed department and IHS reflected attempts by the federal government to prioritize public health care services for all Canadians—including Indian people. Under this new bureaucratic regime, Indian Affairs was no longer directly responsible for Indian health care.[7]

The director of Indian Health Services throughout most of this period (1946–65) was Dr. Percy E. Moore. A native of Ontario, he was a graduate of the University of Manitoba medical school and a specialist in public health. Moore had some experience working as medical superintendant of the Fisher River Indian Agency in Manitoba prior to his appointment as director of IHS. When he started work, Moore was immediately confronted with two main difficulties in his role as IHS director. First and foremost, he had to address the tuberculosis crisis

and related poor health conditions in Canada's Aboriginal population, which had some of the highest mortality and morbidity rates
in the country. Second, he inherited a system in which the various
Christian churches played a significant role in Aboriginal health care.
In Moore's view, the Church-run facilities were an "obstacle to the
implementation of a progressive health care system" because he
believed the churches' health care initiatives were too generalized
and were frequently hampered by inter-church competition and pros-
elytizing goals.[8]

Having determined that the health care provided to Indian
peoples was in desperate need of improvement and drawing on his
training in public health, Moore mounted an aggressive campaign to
create a totally secular system of health care facilities to replace those
provided by the churches. His field campaign especially targeted the
areas of Canada where the health of Indian people was deemed most
problematic—particularly those communities in remote and northern
locations in northwestern Canada. For decades, TB had devastated
these Aboriginal communities. As perhaps the single most significant
health challenge, TB directly spurred the formation of formal, state-
operated, health care systems.

Moore's plan of attack was to create facilities ranging from small
nursing outposts to full-service hospitals. To this end, he purchased
decommissioned military hospitals to convert into tuberculosis sanatoria for Aboriginal patients, mobilized resources to create X-ray
patrols and nursing stations, and implemented a program to vac-
cinate all Aboriginal patients demonstrating exposure to TB with the
controversial Bacillus Calmette-Guérin (BCG) vaccine that at the time
had only been selectively used in southern Canada.[9]

Through Moore's efforts, and as part of the national concern
with Indian and Inuit health and its impact on the non-Aboriginal
population, the number of IHS hospitals operated directly by the
Department of National Health and Welfare grew from 17 to 21
between 1945 and 1950.[10] Funding also grew: in 1937 Parliament
voted $750,000 for the medical branch of Indian Affairs; by 1948 that

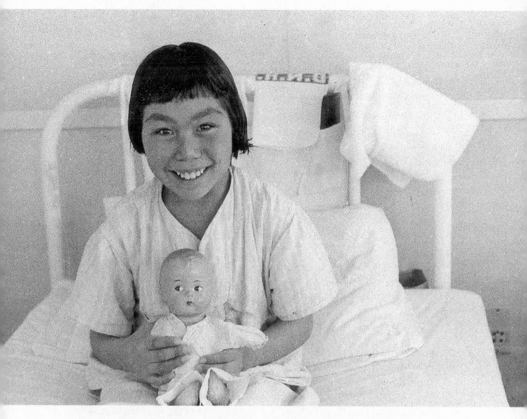

A young girl holds her doll in bed while a patient at the Charles Camsell Indian Hospital, Edmonton, in the 1950s. Federal officials took publicity photographs in the Indian hospitals to demonstrate the effectiveness of the medical service it was providing First Nations and Inuit. These same photographs, and others taken by hospital staff, were used to illustrate an annual yearbook for patients in the hospital, the Charles Camsell Indian Hospital *Pictorial Review*, showing life at the hospital in a given year. [PAA 91.383.79]

amount increased to $7,500,000.[11] Although other mission and public hospitals were also available to First Nations, the IHS institutions were specifically for registered Indian and Inuit patients. Of all Indian hospitals within the IHS, the largest were located in British Columbia and Alberta. In 1946 the Nanaimo Indian Hospital consisted of 210 beds, while the larger Charles Camsell Hospital initially offered 350 and grew quickly to over 500 by 1952.[12]

In his zeal to improve Aboriginal health, Dr. Moore took a bold step that would dramatically affect Aboriginal patients with far-reaching cultural and social consequences—he insisted that northern tuberculosis patients receive treatment in the South and vigorously opposed the creation of sanatoria in the North. His reasoning, based on research that revealed that hospitals in the North had too many empty beds, was intended to make hospitals more efficient. According to Dr. G.J. Wherrett's findings from a 1945 investigation in the Northwest Territories funded through a special Rockefeller Foundation grant, the churches and their facilities were failing. Wherrett described a surfeit of hospital beds in the North available to Aboriginal people and a scarcity in the South:

> The hospitals are mainly operated in the Territories by the missions of both the Church of England in Canada and the Roman Catholic Church. This applies to the two hospitals at Aklavik and the hospitals at Fort Simpson, Fort Resolution, Fort Rae and Fort Smith....The Indian Affairs Branch now operates the hospital at Fort Norman. The mining companies own and operate the hospital at Yellowknife....The Government of Canada has contributed towards the construction costs of some of the mission hospitals and also pays a fixed amount per day for each native, indigent white or half-breed receiving treatment....One is amazed at the number of hospital beds which are to be found in the Mackenzie River area and appalled at what little use is made of them. In the Yukon and the North West Territories, the ratio of hospital beds per 1,000 population (30.1) is four times that of British Columbia, which has the highest hospital bed complement of all the provinces.... When these hospitals were visited they were practically empty.[13]

Wherrett described high death rates among northern indigenous peoples, shortages of medical personnel and equipment, as well as the government's ad hoc approach to medical services in the North. Strongly reacting to Wherrett's report, Moore uncompromisingly developed a plan to move Aboriginal health care south—a move that today seems contrary to the logic of keeping northern hospital beds open for Aboriginal patients close to their local communities and enhancing hospital facilities in southern Canada.

As a result of his plan, patients—especially the TB patients—were removed from their northern home communities to the distant South to receive treatments. Many had never travelled outside of their local

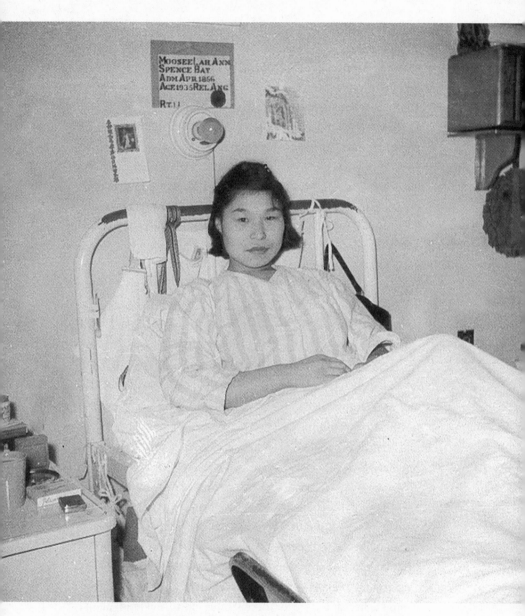

A patient from Spence Bay, NWT, on bed rest at the Charles Camsell Indian Hospital, Edmonton, 1950s. Patients had little personal space in the large hospital wards; a nightstand held personal items such as clothing, cigarettes, and letters, while a nearby shelf housed the popular radio. [PAA 91.383.85]

environs. Many never returned. This loss of relatives and close family members, both young and old, devastated the small northern communities infected by tuberculosis and other diseases. For decades, Dr. Moore's steadfast decision had deep and lasting impact on Aboriginal communities.

Examining the Canadian government's perspective on Aboriginal peoples throws light on Moore's success in initiating his plan. Significantly, decision-making for IHS followed hierarchical lines. Many employees in the system had served in the military during the Second World War and were familiar with that kind of structure. Everyone—from politicians and bureaucrats to caregivers—were primarily urbanites. Indian health policy was devised first and foremost in Ottawa, far from the realities of the "bush" life. In fact, those working out in the field for the IHS bureaucracy referred jokingly to the Department of National Health and Welfare as the department of "wealth and hellfare,"[14] since the bureaucracy was often out of touch with local situations. Despite this distance, the government was clear about its mission. Aboriginal health care was in crisis and the federal government considered itself morally responsible to correct and thus resolve "the problem" of Aboriginal people by promoting health, assimilation, eradication of traditional medical practices, and removing the threat of spreading epidemics to non-Aboriginal populations.

Indian Health Services had four strategic goals worth noting. Taken together these goals showed a conspicuous absence of any notions of self-determination or autonomy in health care for First Nations. The federal government would take care of Indian and Inuit health, not the Aboriginal peoples themselves.

First and foremost among its goals, IHS sought "to provide a complete health service for these [Status Indian and Inuit] peoples" based on a moral, not a legal, imperative. More directly, "Canada's Indian Health Service...has arisen, not from legislative obligation, but rather as a moral undertaking to succour the less fortunate and to raise the standard of health generally."[15]

A second goal was to "improve assimilation" of Indian peoples into mainstream non-Native society. Healthy Indian people were deemed to be more economically independent and less dependent on government, and thus better able to join Canada as workers rather than wards.[16]

Third, there was no support for nor understanding of traditional Aboriginal health practices. Until at least the 1960s, traditional medicines and practices were viewed as backwards, and based on superstition and ignorance. The aim of IHS was to "correct" the traditional medical and health practices of Aboriginal peoples: "It is not as if we were merely trying to replace ignorance with correct attitudes and knowledge. We are trying to introduce new attitudes and practices to people who already have strong feelings and traditions about sickness and its treatment, however erroneous these may be.[17]

Fourth, IHS made it clear that its primary interest was public health: "Public health education and practice has been the keynote of Indian Health Services, the avowed purpose being to forestall disease and detect it in the earliest stages."[18] This was not a surprising priority given that tuberculosis among Aboriginal peoples at this time had an incidence rate more than ten times that of the non-Aboriginal Canadian population. In the eyes of government officials and health workers, this represented a significant public health threat to non-Aboriginal Canadians in the southern regions of Canada.[19] In fact, tuberculosis rates were so high that in 1951–52 tuberculosis patients occupied 75 per cent of IHS hospital beds.[20]

In keeping with these goals and ideals, IHS operated hospitals, nursing stations, health centres, clinics, and special travelling clinics mobilized by IHS boats and buses, and employed an army of medical officers and nurses to staff them. Commitment to the creation and expansion of IHS increased rather dramatically in the two and a half decades of the postwar years. The IHS annual report for 1946–47 records that there were 18 hospitals and 22 nursing stations (not including health centres or clinics) staffed by 119 field and hospital workers. By 1961–62 the annual report counted 19 IHS hospitals and 43 nursing stations staffed by 696 workers (see Appendix One). Funding for IHS and its staffing and facilities also grew over time, showing the most growth between 1946 and the mid-1960s (see Appendix Two).

The hospitals operated by IHS varied in size, from four to over three hundred beds. Some of these hospitals were old military facilities, others former mission hospitals, and some were built specifically as Indian hospitals in the era prior to the creation of Indian Health Services.[21] The hospitals would serve as the main hubs in the delivery of formal health care to Indian and Inuit people. In communities where IHS supported larger and more sophisticated hospital facilities, doctors and nurses were responsible for patient care as well as serving the local community. In the small city of Nanaimo on Vancouver Island, for example, the Nanaimo Indian Hospital took patients from all northwest coastal First Nations communities. It also served as an important base for doctors working on local reserves or in residential schools.

Despite the growth in health care facilities—including nursing stations, clinics, and health centres after the war—the federal government was never keen on maintaining them. From the start, the federal government was always interested in sharing its care of Aboriginal patients with the provinces and the churches. Surprisingly, its implied aim, as repeatedly stated in the annual reports, was to avoid the creation of a separate health care system for either registered Indian peoples or other Aboriginal groups: "Over and above the facilities operated by the Indian Health Services, arrangements are made for the treatment of persons of native status at several hundreds of general and special hospitals. These include the foremost teaching institutions, community hospitals and a number of mission hospitals whose clientele is almost exclusively Indian and Eskimo....In several provinces the provincial health nursing service extends to native groups, a most happy arrangement which wipes out any feeling of distinction between racial groups."[22]

Indian people and Inuit who did not have direct access to IHS facilities were able to seek treatment at private and community hospitals, which were subsidized by the federal government in exchange for taking these patients. The aim was that eventually Indian and other Aboriginal communities would take over their own service delivery. The 1953 annual report claimed: "As groups become able to obtain these services through their own resources, they are encouraged to do so."[23]

The British Columbia situation was unique in the country. Unlike in other places in Canada, a cost-sharing agreement was worked out between the federal government and the province regarding payment for government medical services provided to Indian people. Starting in 1949, the Canadian government contributed to BC's Hospital Insurance Plan on behalf of Indian people. Registered Indian people in British Columbia received health care from a variety of sources: Church hospitals and nursing stations, as well as IHS-run hospitals in places like Miller Bay in Prince Rupert and the Nanaimo Indian Hospital.

IHS enthusiastically endorsed this position as aligning with its avowed goals: "What will undoubtedly prove to be one of the most outstanding advances in the history of native health was made when the Indians of British Columbia were included in the Hospital Insurance Plan, which came into effect on January 1, 1949. Not only will this facilitate hospital arrangements in that province, but it is a major step in the social and economic development of these people."[24]

Medical Services Branch, 1962–1970s

Although IHS's administration was in Ottawa, its bureaucratic structure changed a number of times between 1945 and the 1970s. In 1962 IHS was reorganized and subsumed under the auspices of a new federal governmental branch called Medical Services, which represented the amalgamation of several federal medical service arms for Canadians outside the domain of provincial programs.

In the 1960s Canada was subdivided into five regions, which served as administrative units, and twenty-two zones, each with its own administrative office. At that time, as part of the Medical Services branch, the IHS director, Dr. Moore, still controlled medical services in regions and zones across Canada.[25]

The purpose of this system appears to have been to deal with different health care needs of various Aboriginal communities. The federal government recognized that local decision-making was logical and necessary in northern and western Canada, where patient needs, local landscapes, and government access varied tremendously. It is worth noting that northwestern Canada, including northern Manitoba, Saskatchewan, Alberta, BC, and the Yukon and Northwest Territories, represented four of the five administrative regions. Eastern Canada was subsumed under a single region until 1966—perhaps because the population from this region was perceived as being less needy than the others.[26]

Beginning in the 1960s, the federal government started training Aboriginal people in health and sanitation issues and employed them within their own communities as health aides and sanitation aides. Community health aides were generally local Aboriginal women, who took on first-aid care responsibilities for their communities, and the sanitation aides were local men charged with cleaning up and organizing water supplies and garbage disposal in their areas.

The inspiration to train local people to look after their own interests was partly a result of national interest in "community development," as well as a response to rising frustration among IHS workers who complained, "Telling has not worked."[27] Realizing that health care needed to have community involvement spurred IHS to create training programs that bridged the "cultural gap" between Medical Services personnel and their Aboriginal patients. Made up of community members from various remote locations, the sanitation and health care training programs continued into the early 1970s.

In some communities, IHS attempted to support health and welfare committees, for which an IHS nurse would serve as secretary. Medical Services hoped that such committees or community groups would gradually take on more responsibility for local health care. In Saskatchewan, IHS staff was cautiously optimistic about this idea, commenting in 1960: "The idea of Committees is still relatively new in Saskatchewan and we must not expect too much in the way of results....Certainly there seems to be a slowly spreading general trend amongst the Indians to want more responsibilities. Our main job in this line is to be ready to take every opportunity towards training them to be able to handle the tasks they want to do."[28]

In this way, IHS, and later Medical Services, slowly devolved responsibilities for health care delivery to local Aboriginal communities even as it maintained control over that care's form and nature.

Dismantling the System, 1970s Onward

Although unwilling to invest too much in permanent health care, the federal government continued expanding IHS facilities and staffing until the early 1970s. After that time, government restructuring, the emergence of universal health care, a declining need for tuberculosis control, and the devolution of health care responsibilities to First Nations themselves—as notions of self-determination gained traction—all contributed to an altered federal involvement in Aboriginal health care.

The beginning of medical insurance in Canada dramatically curbed the federal government's commitment to Indian health. As medical historian T. Kue Young notes, "With the removal of financial barriers to health care, the problem of Indian health services was deemed by many to be solved."[29] Only nursing stations were consistently viewed as the foundation of the system. These facilities, serving Aboriginal peoples directly, remained concentrated in more remote and northern areas.[30]

The Indian Hospital system in Canada was gradually dismantled starting in the 1970s, as need for tuberculosis treatment declined. This was also a time when First Nations communities increasingly began demanding self-governance and self-administration of many of the services—including health services—which had been controlled by the federal government up until that time. By 1985 the Department of National Health and Welfare established the Sub-committee on the Transfer of Health Programs to Indian Control; by 1986 discussions between the federal government and band governments to guide the process of health program transfer to band control began.[31] The peak of the federally controlled Indian Hospital system was thus in the postwar period, through the 1950s and into the early 1970s.

Of course the hospitals did not all shut down at once. Rather, in some areas these institutions were maintained as long as possible for lack of any other appropriate services to replace them, or until they could be transferred to territorial or provincial control.[32] In the 1980s, a flurry of construction saw the creation of new federal nursing stations and health centres to replace the shrinking hospital numbers. By the late 1980s, the Medical Services branch operated only eight hospitals. At the same time it maintained five hundred other health facilities of a smaller nature, with the intention of "getting out of the hospital business."[33]

Overall, it might be said that Canada's federal involvement in Indian health care delivery and administration has moved through a cycle of being based in ideas of "moral imagination"[34] or "helping" to notions of "self-determination." Initially, the federal government firmly rooted its involvement in health care in a sense of moral duty, and the practice of formal health care delivery was based on the idea that Aboriginal peoples needed a helping hand to improve their health conditions because they were unable to help themselves. The result, for a large part of the twentieth century, was a type of health care emphasizing social and cultural change for the supposed "betterment" of the health of Indian and Inuit communities. By the late 1960s, such ideas gradually began to wane as Aboriginal peoples began insisting on the right to determine for themselves what type of care and services most benefitted their communities. This emergence of self-determination in health care, of course, ran parallel to self-determination in education and politics so prominent in public conversation between Aboriginal peoples and the federal government. After the 1970s, the devolution of health care practice and decision-making gradually moved more and more into the hands of

Aboriginal peoples themselves, although the professions responsible for implementing health care policy and practices remained primarily non-Aboriginal until more recently. The struggle to reclaim indigenous notions of health and health care is ongoing today.

NURSING WORK AT THE UNITED CHURCH HOSPITAL, BELLA BELLA, BRITISH COLUMBIA

Marge Thompson

In May 1976 Joy Duncan interviewed Marge Thompson as part of Duncan's Frontier Nursing Project (1911–76) in Sardis, BC. Thompson's work at the United Church hospital in Bella Bella marked the start of her work with Aboriginal communities. Although she began her career in a mission hospital, she later moved on to the Indian Health Services' Miller Bay Indian Hospital in Prince Rupert, BC. Many of her patients had tuberculosis. As a nurse working in a remote location, her duties were varied, and she worked both in and outside the hospital. This narrative is an adaptation of an interview held in the Glenbow Archives fonds entitled: "Joy Duncan's Frontier Nursing Project, 1974–1978," interview with Marge Thompson.

I WAS BORN IN QUEBEC and attended school and university in Saskatchewan. I completed my nurse's training at the Vancouver General Hospital. In 1939 I took a position at the Bella Bella Hospital, three hundred miles from Vancouver, run by the United Church. I was inspired by Dr. Grenfell, the doctor who pioneered the outpost hospitals in Labrador, and after I heard him speak on the radio I took the position.

It was a hospital that was amazingly well supplied. In fact, it was a training school until 1936. Students trained for two years at Bella Bella and then one year at the Vancouver General Hospital. It was good training. I did a lot of surgery at the hospital. We had five nurses who provided 24-hour coverage for 20 or 25 patients, although during the war there were often 40 patients. After the war, nurses were very scarce. In the early 1940s an air base was built at Bella Bella and this brought hundreds of airmen and their wives, who were all pregnant, to the community. So we recruited Native girls to work with us, to help with general chores. We gave them on-the-job training. Two-thirds of the patients were Native.

The Church did not support the hospital financially. In 1949 BC's Hospital Insurance system came in, which paid for Indian patients. Before that, the federal government paid $2.50 per day for the Indians.

I was the matron at the hospital until it closed in 1951 and stayed in Bella Bella until 1958. Even though I worked in the hospital, the work was also public health nursing. I made house calls and did prenatal checks in the outpatient department. We knew the patients and things about them. It was a very broad nursing experience.

It was frustrating but rewarding work. I enjoyed the staff and watching them make progress. Many were outstanding, individually. Many went on to advance their education and have successful careers. Other times you felt like the hospital and its buildings were old, inadequate, and crowded.

In the 1950s I took a course in hospital organization and management. As a result of that I moved to Prince Rupert to work at the Miller Bay Hospital for the Department of National Health and

Welfare. In that job I visited reserves as a public health nurse. I didn't feel like I was helping make any change. I visited many places, but there was little change.

NURSING WORK AT THE ANGLICAN HOSPITALS IN AKLAVIK AND PANGNIRTUNG

Biddy Worsley

Biddy Worsley worked for several years at the All Saints Anglican Hospital in Aklavik, a Church hospital funded by the federal government's Indian Affairs branch in the 1940s, and later by Indian Health Services. Remarkably, this was one of the few hospitals that participated in training Aboriginal women as nurse aides and ward maids in the 1940s in the hopes of improving community health in the region.

Her account shows the perspective of a nurse working in one of the subsidized hospitals, remote from Canada's larger urban health care facilities. Worsley also worked in other federal health care centres serving Indian peoples, including the tuberculosis facility at Mill Bay on Vancouver Island, BC, and the Anglican hospital at Pangnirtung on Baffin Island in Canada's far North.

In 1976 Joy Duncan interviewed Biddy Worsley in Duncan on Vancouver Island, BC, as part of the Frontier Nursing Project (1911–76). This narrative is an adaptation of an interview held in the Glenbow

Archives in Calgary, Alberta, under the fonds entitled:
"Joy Duncan's Frontier Nursing Project, 1974–1978," interview with
Biddy Worsley.

~~~~~~~~~~~~~~~~~~

I WORKED AT THE SOLARIUM at Mill Bay before going north.
I received a letter from a girl I knew in Saskatchewan saying they
needed a nurse at the Anglican Mission, so I decided to go. I wasn't
sure at first if this was the right thing for me to do, but my friend
wrote to me and said, "I hope it will be the will of God that you will
see your way to do this." So I prayed for three weeks. After that I was
sure.

There was no orientation for us before going. I first flew to
Edmonton, then to Norman Wells, and finally on to Aklavik. I arrived
there in the summer, July 1954. I don't think I had any preconceived
ideas about the place, but it was a bit of a shock to arrive there. The
community was maybe one thousand to two thousand people. About
half of those were Indian and the other half Eskimo. Aklavik was a
naval base so there were quite a few white people.

The hospital was not fancy. It wasn't modern. We had the basics
but there was no water supply or sewage system. In the winter we
had to be so careful with water, which we pumped up from the
river. We also used ice blocks in the winter. There were about one
hundred beds, and most were filled with long-term tuberculosis
patients. Tuberculosis had decimated the population in that area in
the 1940s and 1950s. The rest of the hospital's patients were children
and maternity cases. There were two doctors, who were employed
by the federal government. The living accommodations were nice
enough—I had my own room.

I was never lonely up there. There were enough white people in
the settlement for visiting back and forth. I went on hikes, walks,
played games, read books, and I enjoyed photography. I was raised in
the country, so I didn't mind being away from a city. I did feel a little
cut off or isolated at first because I was used to having a car, and now

I didn't have one. And I did feel a little removed from the centre of the world. I was now way out on the perimeter and wondered what was happening. I was missing it. And then the longer I was North, I was in the centre of my world again, and the "outside" or down South became "outside." It was not the centre of my world anymore—I was the centre of my world. There were a group of nurses at the hospital and we had lots of fun. We had mail once a week, and we shopped by catalogue.

We didn't really socialize with the Natives, but I did learn a lot about them. I was impressed by their openness. Quite early on, on the first or second day I was in Aklavik, somebody came up to me on the street and shook my hand. They said, "Welcome to Aklavik." It was an Indian or an Eskimo. I was really surprised. And being a nurse in the hospital and having all these Native patients, I couldn't fail but to get to know them as people. And this was really exciting for me—you know, to be in the midst of another culture. It was sort of marvellous. I was lucky enough to be doing a job that was needed. It was interesting, useful, and enjoyable work. That, plus meeting all these wonderful people.

It was a very, very happy situation. We white people were in the minority. It was their place and that made all the difference in the world. We were the guests, the intruders. We were useful but it was their place and that makes all the difference. So I don't think there was a lot of resentment towards the white people at the time I was there. Or I would say hardly any resentment that I was aware of. Unless I was totally unaware or unless we were particularly fortunate in the hospital. They were very friendly, open, welcoming, appreciative and had so many qualities to admire, like dignity and resourcefulness.

In 1961 the All Saints Hospital closed. So I moved to a small Anglican hospital at Pangnirtung on Baffin Island. It was a thirty-bed hospital. Over half of the patients had tuberculosis. There were Eskimo girls who helped at the hospital, and we were in the minority again. Most of the staff at the hospital were Eskimo, not white. We employed Eskimo. We weren't immersed in Eskimo culture, but we weren't separate either because we were very dependent on them, very dependent, which is good. Several Eskimos worked for us. Sometimes there were more Indian and Eskimo than white staff at the hospital. So if they all walked out the door or got sick at the same time we'd be devastated. This is great. It was interdependence. They were resourceful, proud, independent people that appreciated the medical thing. I know it's not like this everywhere.

DIRECTOR OF NURSING AT THE CAMSELL
Elva Taylor

In October 1991 Lisa Staples interviewed Elva Taylor as part of a project documenting Charles Camsell Indian Hospital history.[1] As a former director of nursing for the hospital, and as president of the Charles Camsell Historical Society, Elva Taylor was eager to help reveal important aspects of hospital life, especially the extensive handicraft program run by the hospital's Occupational Therapy Department.

Taylor served at the Camsell for many years, and as director of nursing she was instrumental in hiring and training many Native people in health care work at the hospital. She encouraged many young Aboriginal women to work as nurses' aides and perhaps consider careers in nursing work. Her enthusiasm for her work and the handicraft program is reflected in the interview. She believed that hospital treatment in Edmonton was the best solution to the tuberculosis crisis.

Although Elva Taylor's memories were recorded to highlight the history of the occupational therapy arts and crafts program they also give a feeling for the responsibility that nurses like Taylor felt to make things "better" for Aboriginal peoples. Her memories reflect the social hierarchy in institutions like hospitals at this time, where patients were "wards" and the staff had a great deal of authority over a patient's life, despite language and cultural barriers.

Although hospital life was difficult for patients, in Elva Taylor's view, at least it taught them new lessons. She believed it offered patients new job opportunities and a new education. Taylor didn't seem to question her own authority nor that of the hospital to work as it did: determining the lives of patients.

~~~~~~~~~~~~~~~~~~~~~

I STARTED THE 8TH OF DECEMBER 1947, and I finished at the end of August 1971, and then transferred to Canada Manpower as a counsellor. But, all the years at Camsell my position was director of nursing. It was a real experience. I liked it very much; it was very interesting, and a challenge. We had wonderful staff and the patients were wonderful as you got to know them and they got to know us. It was a real experience.

Well, the hospital had been operating almost two years when I went there so I learned about the answers to your question from some of the staff that had been there. The very first people transferred from the TB ward at the Edmonton General were Native people.

When they first came in it was a very foreign experience for many of them, particularly if they were from the northern part of Alberta. The southern people from Cardston, and the Blackfoot at Gleichen, they had little hospitals there so it wasn't so foreign. But to come and be with people who were from other areas or reserves was a great difference for them.

There was a problem with language among one another and with us. We tried to get around communication gaps and barriers

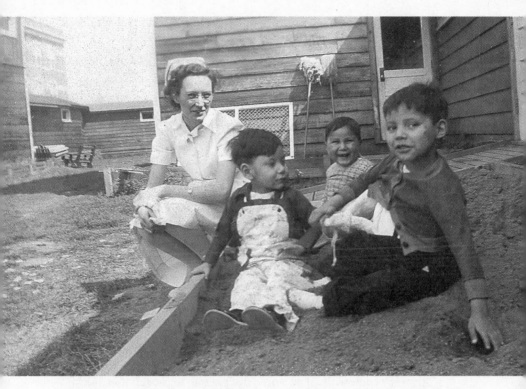

Elva Taylor, RN, director of nursing, in a sandbox with young patients at the Charles Camsell Hospital, 1950s. [PAA 91.383.146]

pretty much with pantomime, gestures, and showing them the item you were wanting to describe or wanting them to use. If there was someone who was fluent in their own language and could speak some English you could use them as interpreters. So there were a variety of ways that we tried to do it. They were very good.

I always remember when I asked a lady to interpret for me for a woman who was in labour. The lady who was in labour made a sign to the lady who was doing the interpreting—from her mouth, back to the lady, and then back to her own ear. I asked the interpreter what did she mean by this? What she meant was, "Words from her mouth don't mean anything to my ears." But I wouldn't have been able to determine this, but this other Native lady could even though she couldn't really make her understand. As I say, a lot of it was gestures, facial expressions.

We had teachers very early, and the teachers paid no attention as to the age of a person. If the person was interested in education then they were able to receive whatever they could assimilate or were interested in. If the people were interested the teachers would teach. This made a great difference. Some of these older people who were parents saw the need for education for their children and grandchildren. When they went home, the parents promoted education.

Patients were interested education, but it would depend, and some of them were so lonely it would take quite a while for them to adjust and become interested. It took time sometimes to find what they were interested in, in the way of occupational therapy or in education. Some wanted to learn to write their own name, others wanted to learn to read. Another place they got some ideas of language and customs outside of their own areas, whether it was good or bad, were the picture shows we used to show.

In the very beginning they were Indian patients. The idea was to get the people with far advanced disease into the hospital as quickly as possible to try and stop the spread of tuberculosis among the people at home. As that was accomplished in the southern part and central part of the province, the authorities began to accept patients from the North, the Yukon, and then the Territories.

The Inuit people were actually apprehensive and fearful of the Indian people. I think that dates back to the massacre that took place at Coppermine, many, many years ago. Some of the northern Indian people in that area actually murdered some of the Eskimo people.

They were very reserved, the Inuit people. We did forsake of custom and language—the Inuit people have a common language but different dialects—but we would do our very best to put them together, and if there were just two in one room we put them together; we would put them in bed side by side so they could communicate with one another. With the older people who didn't know English, if there was a younger person from their area who had disease that was such that they could be together we did that, too. It's

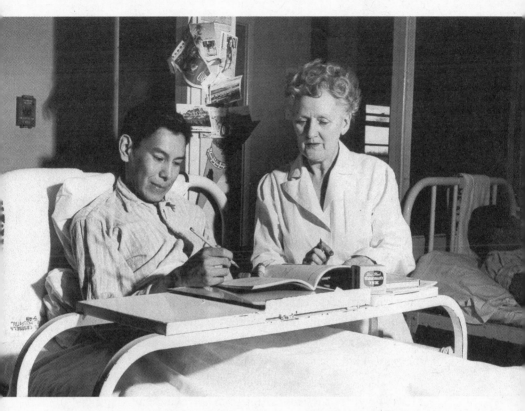

Patient and teacher engaging in schoolwork, Charles Camsell Indian Hospital, 1950s. It was not uncommon for students from Indian Residential Schools to contract tuberculosis while at school. Their studies were not stopped during their stay in the hospital, however, as the Department of Indian Affairs provided teachers in the Indian Hospital system. [PAA 91.383.58]

just like being isolated when no matter how many people are around you you're not able to communicate.

One of the things about the Eskimo people was that we always found they were cheerful and pleasant. They figured that was the way they were expected to appear to us. There were so many things that we didn't understand about one another. Many, many things.

In recent months I've come to think of the Camsell Hospital as being more of a college than a hospital. With what the patients learned from one another and about one another, plus their education, plus what they learned about health, you add all this together, and to me, I think of it now as college. When I think of how many of them went home and became leaders in their own communities, and certainly now beyond their own communities.

Abraham Okpik was a patient; he was there when I got there and was discharged not long after he became the first Inuit representative on the Northwest Territories council. There was a measles epidemic at Aklavik at the end of 1948, and we sent three nurses and they set up a hospital in school and Abraham was their nursing orderly. From what he learned when he was a patient at the Camsell he just knew how to fit in and was able to help them and he was part of the staff.

We often hired a number of people that had been patients as orderlies and nursing aides. Sometimes wives would work on staff while their husbands were patients in the hospital. And Mr. Noel was one of the first of the Indian men to be on the janitorial staff while his wife was a patient. This was informal policy at first, but later we had requests from Ottawa to try to give employment to them, but that was an informal thing and a humanitarian thing.

We also set up an arrangement with the Department of Indian Affairs for girls on the reserve interested in taking a nursing aides course, which at that time was given in Calgary. When the girls graduated they were certified nursing aides. They would come to the Camsell for a two-month assessment so they would learn something about hospitals and find out whether or not they truly would be interested in that kind of work. This was part of our work, to assess them.

The people we felt would manage to cope with this kind of a program and most likely be successful would be recommended back to the Department of Indian Affairs, who was responsible for that kind of education, and they would go to the nursing aide school. I don't know if any of the girls who became nursing aides became nurses but certainly some of the Native girls became nurses and some of them were on our staff.

Many people purchased crafts from the occupational therapy program. Some of the customers were friends of the staff, [and] later, people who lived near to the hospital or people from service clubs would come and buy. They got us to make small souvenirs for conventions and there would be things that we would try and make. It was principally people who came to visit, and word of mouth. We never advertised. If you heard of someone wanting something of the sort then they would go to the gift shop. The hospital was the only source of crafts around here.

It was the men who did the carving. I'm not sure about the wood carving whether they did that or not when Mr. Lord started the program. The more I think about it, I think he was responsible for getting the soapstone carving underway. Prior to this it was probably leatherwork that they did.

The soapstone would have had to be shipped in. It seemed to me there must have been some from Coppermine way. There were remarks on the inferiority of Quebec soapstone and better quality from Coppermine. It may have been that there would have been chunks brought in by people coming down.

A lot of them did very nice work. I don't have a lot of soapstone but I have one wooden carving from David Koomiak from Victoria Island/Cambridge Bay area, and his wood carvings were beautiful. As far as I know he only carved in wood. He did a face of an Eskimo with parka and fur, and Dr. Green purchased that one.

I would suspect he started at the hospital because he was fairly young when he was admitted so I would think he learned at the hospital. I know the last time he was in hospital was in 1971 for his check up. Dr. Gray didn't think that he would be able to go home because of his bilateral prostheses (his feet), so he arranged for David to work at the hospital. David worked with the laundry and the linen supply.

Finally one day David told the doctor that he needed to go home and kill polar bears. When I saw him later in 1971 he had killed five polar bears and his partner killed four polar bears. He walked; he didn't use canes. When he went back north, he was the handy-man at the nursing station at Cambridge Bay. It was "the call of the North" for David. This was true for most of our patients, for the far northern people and the Indian people.

Well, it was hard for some of the patients. Some of them were in for a long time, and yet on the other hand if we hadn't brought them out they wouldn't have lived and the tuberculosis would never have been brought under control. For us, if we had tuberculosis, back when I was a child, we'd have to go miles from home to a sanatorium. While it seems very unkind, what is the most unkind? To let the disease spread? Or to take these people and bring them to a centre where they would get really good care? The mission hospitals throughout the North were utilized for a period of time to try to assist with the control of the spread and get people into a hospital setting.

3

THE INSTITUTIONS
Indian Hospitals and Field Nursing

House of Commons, Ottawa, 1951:
Mr. Martin, Minister of Health and Welfare: In addition to our 18 hospitals—
those at Qu'Appelle, at Nanaimo, at Coqualeetza and the Charles Camsell hospital
are the major ones—we have 29 nursing stations and 49 health centres.

House of Commons, Ottawa, 1952:
Mr. Martin, Minister of Health and Welfare: The Indian hospitals are good hospitals. There is no over-extravagance. They are not comparable in some respects
with the material set-up of corresponding institutions, although service is good
and is one that this country can be proud of, in keeping with its duty.[1]

THE IHS SYSTEM OF HOSPITALS and field stations played a profound
role in the lives of First Nations and Inuit patients, their families, and
communities. Operating under the control of Indian Health Services,
these large facilities extended their reach far into the remote North
and West of Canada to grapple with the TB crisis in the small and
remote Arctic, subarctic, and northern communities.

The influence of the IHS hospitals and field system affected Aboriginal people in numerous ways. As part of this program, IHS had a powerful hand in the relocation and re-education of Aboriginal people. Not only that, but IHS also influenced, positively or negatively, the establishment of Aboriginal health care "para-professionals" accredited within that formal health care system. Furthermore, it continued to hold close control over formal health care. A key feature of Canada's IHS service, in contrast with its counterpart in the United States, was an entrenched bureaucratic culture of centralized decision-making—IHS was noteworthy for its not eliciting Aboriginal participation. For the most part, Aboriginal peoples filled service roles within the health care system, not decision-making roles. Administration and delivery of health care services were not devolved to Aboriginal communities. Finally, the hospitals and the field system brought particular treatments to Aboriginal communities; they also confined Aboriginal peoples in the facilities to receive the treatment.

Indian Health Services (and later Medical Services) in the 1950s and 1960s focused on disease prevention and did little to offer communities much beyond non-Native nursing service and hospital care. According to the 1951–52 Department of National Health and Welfare annual report: "Public health education and practice has been the keynote of Indian Health Services, the avowed purpose being to forestall disease or detect it in the earliest stages. [When illness was inevitable,] the patients have been either admitted to departmental treatment facilities or arrangements made for care by the professional and hospital services in the communities close by the patients' homes."[2]

As a result, the services promoted health education, immunization programs, and extensive health surveys for prevention and early detection. Most important, they also supported the building and use of a large number of hospitals, ranging from small remote facilities to full-service institutions based in urban centres. It was the hospitals that were considered the centrepiece of the services.

The hospital experience touched the lives of both the sick and the healthy, and represented a force of change in many Aboriginal communities. As they received treatment for tuberculosis, Aboriginal patients resided for long periods of time in IHS hospitals, and consequently their families and communities became tied to the institutions directly and indirectly. Unlike in IHS health centres and nursing outposts, patients who entered into the hospital system generally stayed for at least a few months. In addition, through the various education and rehabilitation programs offered within these facilities, the future lives and careers of many patients were further influenced. Although many patients were able to return home once they experienced a remission in their tuberculosis, others found themselves unable to reconnect with their families or communities after experiencing such a lengthy illness. As a result of education and work experience gained within the Indian hospital, or new friends and family acquired in the institution, some patients found their lives moving in unexpected directions once they regained their health.

Canada's Indian Hospitals

The Department of Indian Affairs and, later, IHS operated a system of hospitals specifically to meet the needs of Canada's registered Indian and Inuit populations. Between the end of the Second World War and the 1970s, these institutions worked in partnership with remote and scattered nursing outposts and health centres to bring formal health care services to Aboriginal communities that previously lacked access to such care. A guiding principle in this system was that hospital services should be as centralized as possible. Tuberculosis control was the system's main priority—especially in northwestern and western Arctic Canada, where Aboriginal communities were devastated by TB, suffering infection rates higher than in eastern and central Canada.[3]

But IHS did not simply manage its own, strictly federal, facilities— it also networked other provincial, charitable, and Church-run institutions into its loose web of hospitals. In British Columbia, for example, the federal government funded the Hospital Insurance Plan

IHS Indian Hospital Facilities in Western Canada, 1947*

Indian Hospital	Province	Number of Beds
Dynevor Hospital	Manitoba	50
Fisher River Hospital	Manitoba	30
Fort Alexander Hospital	Manitoba	20
Clearwater Lake Hospital	Manitoba	78
Norway House Hospital	Manitoba	22
Fort Qu'Appelle Hospital	Saskatchewan	68
Peigan Hospital	Alberta	10
Sarcee Hospital	Alberta	Unavailable
Morley Hospital	Alberta	13
Blackfoot Hospital	Alberta	40
Charles Camsell Hospital	Alberta	310
Blood Hospital	Alberta	45
Coqualeetza Hospital	British Columbia	200
Nanaimo Hospital	British Columbia	210
Miller Bay Hospital	British Columbia	150

*Data based on Canada, Department of National Health and Welfare, Indian Health Services, Annual Report (1945–46) and (1946–47).

for registered Indian people so that they could attend any appropriate hospital facility. Similarly, in Saskatchewan the IHS reimbursed the provincial health care system for registered Indian people who used its services. In Manitoba, in turn, the Dynevor (Selkirk) and Clearwater (The Pas) facilities ran with the assistance of the Sanatorium Board of Manitoba in 1947.[4] The table above shows the main facilities operated by IHS.

Hospitals in the IHS system varied in size and shape. Some were small four-bed institutions located in old mission buildings, while others were constructed specifically as hospitals. In BC the north coast was serviced by the Miller Bay Indian Hospital, a sizeable institution of 150 beds located in a former military facility. In southern Alberta the Blood Indian Hospital, built as a state of the art facility in 1928, was a two-storey brick building with separate open wards for men and women. It featured the latest in interior appointments, including sterilizer machines and new linoleum on all the floors. In contrast, the Norway House Indian Hospital in northern Manitoba consisted of a decommissioned army base that required extensive renovation to update laundry and power provisions.

At the Moose Factory Hospital, which opened in 1949, equipment or facilities were not even completely installed when the first patients arrived. The desperate need to house patients before the approach of winter drove the staff to host patients on mattresses on the floor until beds could be set up.[5] The Moose Factory Hospital also featured an interesting architecture. From the air, it was shaped like the Cross of Lorraine—a double-barred cross serving as the symbol for many anti-tuberculosis organizations. Intentional or not, the meaning was not lost on medical staff flying in and out of the facility.

Two Facilities: The Nanaimo Indian Hospital and the Charles Camsell Indian Hospital

Of all Indian hospitals in the IHS network, the two largest and most renowned in Canada were located in Alberta and British Columbia: the Nanaimo and Charles Camsell Indian Hospitals. Their strategic locations enabled IHS to offer the highest level of care available to the dispersed First Nations communities on Canada's northwest coast and western subarctic and Arctic. In 1946 the Nanaimo Indian Hospital consisted of 210 beds, while the larger Camsell offered 350, growing quickly to 500 in later years.[6] Unlike some of the smaller hospitals, these two institutions could capably handle long-term care patients, surgeries, and lab and X-ray procedures.

When it was first opened in 1945, the Nanaimo Indian Hospital was intended to serve First Nations communities of Vancouver Island and the central northwest coast. With 210 beds, it was larger than the older Coqualeetza Indian Hospital in Sardis, BC. The hospital occupied a decommissioned military barracks on an old army campsite restructured and reconfigured immediately after the war to begin accepting Indian patients. Michael Dick, a former patient

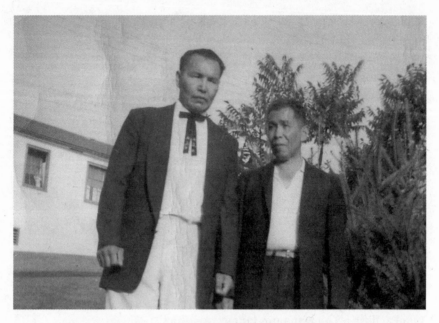

Nanaimo Indian Hospital. Basil Alphonse (left) and friend, 1950s. Few pictures of the Nanaimo Indian Hospital are available. It was popular for family members to take "snaps" of relatives in hospital at this time, and this picture was taken by Mr. Alphonse's daughter, Delores. The hospital is seen in the background. [Delores Louie, private collection]

and later a staff member in the hospital, recalls that when the first patients arrived in the wards, the soldiers were only just leaving.[7]

The hospital was not centrally located within the city but sat up on a hill overlooking Nanaimo. The grounds featured grassy slopes and were partially cleared of forest. From the hilltop, patients and staff had a stunning view of the city and coastline below. Landscaping around the hospital was minimal, and there was no fencing to demarcate hospital property. A large open parking lot sprawled below the barracks buildings.

The buildings consisted of rows of single-storey wooden barracks connected by hallways. Inside, patients occupied "cubicles" consisting of six beds per unit, each cubicle separated by glass wall dividers. Separate wards existed for children, men, and women.[8] In the recollections of those who worked there—or who endured their tuberculosis recovery there—the facilities were basic. In summer, the barracks became insufferably hot when the sun beat relentlessly on the hillside. In winter, radiators worked hard to heat the cubicles and hallways.

Recreational facilities and opportunities in the Nanaimo Indian Hospital were limited. All patients were encouraged to read, work on schoolwork, or do handicrafts if they were able. Leatherwork and sewing were very popular hobbies, and the hospital housed a small library with a few worn paperbacks for patients to borrow. Now and then, someone with a guitar or a radio shared music on a ward. Field trips were rare, but occasionally nurses and doctors took staff and patients on arranged outings down the hill and into the town. Sometimes, to boost the spirit of the patients, staff organized movie nights or scheduled visiting musicians and entertainers to drop by.

Patients in later stages of recovery from TB were allowed outside to enjoy fresh air and visits with friends out-of-doors. Initially, though, patients were not allowed outdoors at all; for in the early years of the hospital's operation many patients were subject to the strictest routines of bed rest employed in all IHS hospitals.[9]

Today, remnants of the hospital's old parking lot remain, but the network of single-storey white clapboard army barracks comprising the actual hospital was demolished in 2004. The site of the Nanaimo Indian Hospital is an empty field overlooking the city of Nanaimo, one with a spectacular view of the Strait of Georgia and the Gulf Islands. Gradually, grass, blackberries, and broom are reclaiming the foundations, which lie behind a barbed-wire fence on Department of National Defence land.

In contrast to the Nanaimo Indian Hospital, the Charles Camsell Indian Hospital was much larger and sophisticated for its time. Considered the veritable "jewel in the crown" of the Indian Health Services hospital system, it was created to serve the prairies, western subarctic, and western Arctic Aboriginal communities.

Originally an old Jesuit College refurbished by the American military during the Second World War, the facility occupied almost an entire city block and was dominated by a central three-storey brick

building. Behind it lay a maze of detached redwood barracks con-
nected to the main building via a long hallway nicknamed the "Burma
Road."[10] Operated by the Americans during their construction of the
Alaska (Alcan) Highway, it was taken over by the Royal Canadian Army
Medical Corps and was known as the Edmonton Military Hospital.

In response to the TB crisis and as a result of growing public
pressure to address the epidemic before it could spread to the
general public, the federal government acted upon the recommendations of the Advisory Committee for the Control and Prevention
of Tuberculosis among the Indians that additional hospitals for TB
treatment be made available.[11] As a result, in June 1946 the Edmonton
Military Hospital was transferred from the Department of National
Defence to the Department of National Health and Welfare as a
TB treatment facility for Indian and Inuit patients. In the summer
of that same year the hospital was renamed the Charles Camsell
Indian Hospital (after a Deputy Minister of Mines and Resources) and
opened to the first Indian and Inuit patients. Children and adults alike
were treated at the hospital. With a capacity of approximately 397
beds, the Camsell featured staff quarters for as many people.

When it was acquired by the federal government, the hospital
came fully equipped with everything from X-ray and dental facilities, warehouses, a gym, a large laboratory, and drug and operating
rooms to ward kitchens, a central cafeteria ready to feed up to two
thousand people, sterilizers, and fridges. In short, it was a full-service
medical establishment; only laundry facilities were missing.[12]

Larger and more technically endowed than the Nanaimo Hospital,
then Minister of Health Paul Martin claimed that the Charles Camsell
Hospital "is one of the outstanding institutions of its kind devoted
exclusively to the treatment of tuberculosis."[13] It was the largest
IHS hospital in the region and was considered the most significant.
It hosted expertise and facilities unavailable in the middle and far
northern regions of western Canada, where surgery and treatment
facilities were less developed and had very limited staff.

For the next three decades the Camsell was the most prominent
institution involved in TB treatment for Inuit and registered Indian

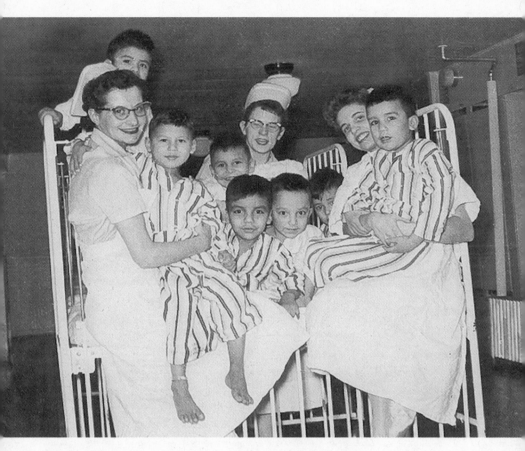

Boys pose with their nurses in the Charles Camsell Indian Hospital,
Edmonton, 1950s. Many Aboriginal children with tuberculosis experienced
lengthy hospital stays, sometimes lasting a number of years.
[PAA 91.383.76]

peoples from the Yukon, Northwest Territories, Northern British
Columbia, and Alberta (whose combined Indian and Inuit population
numbered about 25,700).[14]

Inside the Camsell, Inuit and First Nations patients rested in wards
with few private rooms. In the main building with its multiple storeys,
patients enjoyed opening the windows in summer months, hanging
out into the fresh air and interacting with people on the street below,
much to the chagrin of the medical staff.[15] Other patients were housed

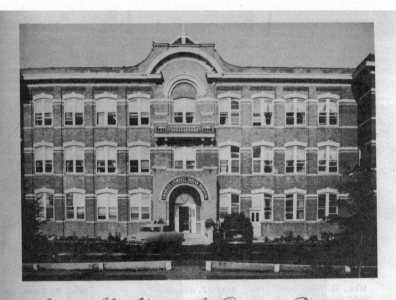

Camsell Hospital Receives Rating

Charles Camsell Hospital operated by the federal department of health for Indian and Eskimo patients, has been fully accredited as a general hospital by the Joint Commission of Accreditation of Hospitals in Chicago.

A representative of the commission inspected the hospital last month and word of the accreditation was received this week by Dr. Matthew Matas, medical superintendent.

The commission is made up of representatives of the American College of Physicians, the American College of Surgeons, the American Hospital Association, the American Medical Association and the Canadian Medical Association.

Originally founded as a tuberculosis hospital, the Camsell Hospital has steadily expanded its facilities until now it has all the facilities of a Grade A general treatment hospital.

1

Charles Camsell Indian Hospital announces its accreditation as a Grade A general treatment hospital. [PAA PR1969.0073/MI] in the various redwood buildings making up the "Camsell complex" behind the old Jesuit college. There, renovations to the original military buildings to turn them into wards tried to keep pace with the influx of patients for the hospital. According to Herbert Roberts, former maintenance supervisor for the Camsell, "As fast as space was created for more beds, it never seemed fast enough, for many times in those early days beds would be set up in the corridors as there was nowhere else to put patients when they arrived in large numbers."[16]

Recreation for patients inside the hospital was offered even if it was limited. Like in the Nanaimo Hospital, bedridden patients were encouraged to listen to bedside radios, play guitar, engage in artwork or handicrafts from their beds, complete schoolwork, or enjoy some of the activities offered through the Occupational Therapy Department within the hospital. As in Nanaimo, the Camsell offered movie nights and various entertainment and performances for its patients. The Camsell also featured a canteen and a gift shop where many patients' craft items were sold. Although the hospital grounds were not extensive and were delimited by a small, white, picket fence, there were small play areas and sandboxes for the children, as well as areas for games like horseshoes for adults. Of course patients did not limit themselves to the official recreation programs—many people recall fondly the practical joking, camaraderie, and horseplay that took place every day on the wards.

At the time it was adopted as a federal government facility, the hospital sat on the edge of Edmonton, in "bush country."[17] In 1965–67 the hospital was rebuilt and enlarged into a fully "modern" facility. The Camsell connected to regional or local provincial health authorities only after 1958, and then only in a minimal way.[18] Modernized and renovated in the mid-1960s, the hospital became a public facility as the city grew around it. Its doors finally closed in 1996. Today, the Charles Camsell Indian Hospital sits empty in Edmonton's northwestern suburb of Inglewood.

Indian Health Services: Activities in the Field

Until the 1960s, IHS kept health care delivery and education in the hands of its almost exclusively non-Native staff, especially the IHS field nurses. As late as 1948–49, Aboriginal communities were still not empowered to self-administer or educate their people as professional or para-professional health care workers. Instead, community education meant "Indian Health Services medical officers and nurses infiltrate into Homemaker Clubs and other women's organizations, giving instructional chats and showing health films,"[19] or "to improve health standards by demonstration, example and gentle pressure."[20] The prevailing attitude was paternalistic, aiming to "show" rather than to "empower" Aboriginal people.

Indian Health Services (and later Medical Services) in the 1950s and 1960s focused on disease prevention. According to annual reports, "Public health education and practice has been the keynote of Indian Health Services, the avowed purpose being to forestall disease or detect it in the earliest stages." When illness was inevitable, "the patients have been either admitted to departmental treatment facilities or arrangements made for care by the professional and hospital services in the communities close by the patients' homes."[21] As a result, the two services promoted health education, immunization programs, and extensive health surveys for prevention and early detection of disease.

In the field, the daily business of Indian Health Services workers included public health nursing, public health education, tuberculosis surveys in Indian residential schools and communities, sanitation surveys, and nursing and hospital treatments. To do this work, IHS employed an army of doctors, nurses, and, by the 1960s, a small group of Aboriginal community health aides and sanitation aides.

IHS nurses were considered the frontline workers. Alone or in teams, they travelled extensively from their nursing outposts or health centres to bring health "education" to Aboriginal communities. Using dogsleds, snowmobiles, boats and canoes, wagons, trucks, snowshoes, and even walking, they worked hard to reach their clients.

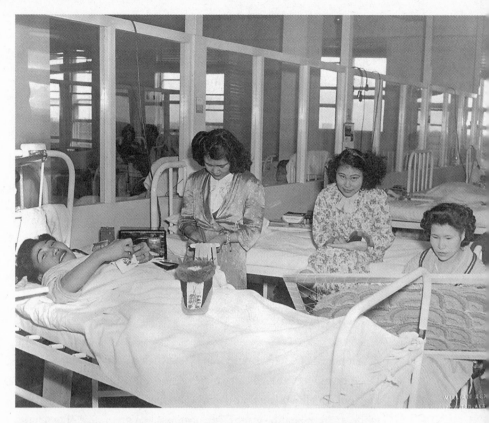

Women's ward, Charles Camsell Indian Hospital, 1950s. Women are working on handicrafts. Note the bedside radio. For many bedridden patients, the opportunity to do craftwork helped them to pass the time as well as earn some spending money for use in the hospital canteen or to buy clothing or craft materials. [PAA 91.383.103]

Official IHS blue parkas, part of their field uniform, announced their presence. In 1961 a formal badge was devised "to provide a device which the Indians and Eskimos will come to recognize as a symbol of help and understanding." The symbol was a large white North Star upon which was placed a red arrow entwined by a golden serpent.[22]

The main messages carried by the nurses included directions for "clean living," proper baby care, good nutrition, and disease prevention. They also brought immunizations. To enhance and further their work, the nurses distributed booklets like *Good Health for Canada's Indians* and *The Book of Wisdom*, created especially for the Inuit.[23] Nurses were also armed with filmstrips, films, and posters. One of the more popular filmstrips in the 1950s was *The Starlight Story*, a full-colour forty-frame strip produced as a joint effort between the National Film Board and Department of National Health and Welfare.

As part of their teaching mission, nurses also worked in Indian day and residential schools where IHS encouraged students to make posters. One long-standing contest ran for more than sixteen years within the Indian Affairs school system; similar poster contests were also held in IHS hospitals. The contests generated such slogans as:

> "Make War on TB!"
> "No TB in our TeePee"
> "No Treaty; Fight TB"
> "Have'm Peace; Conquer TB"
> "Hunt TB: Get a chest X-ray"

Employing posters, books, films, and their own medical training, field nurses were able to carry their version of health care to families and individuals who might otherwise not come into direct contact with Canada's health system. The notion that a great deal of teaching had to be done was common in this period. After using a film projector and generator to teach modern health practices in her remote nursing outpost, one nurse, Mrs. Muriel Schonbert, RN, reported: "Years of patient teaching must take place to change the attitude of isolated people, who, through no fault of their own, are really living a life which can be compared to the dark ages. The film may well prove to be a shortcut."[24]

At their home base, whether a modest nursing outpost or a larger health centre, nurses continued the work of tending to patients confined to bed inside the facility or offering first-aid care to those who came seeking medical help. In this way, nurses treated everything from emergencies to long-term illnesses. Many also took a great deal of time to counsel and support maternity cases, whether prenatal or postnatal, because baby care was a priority.

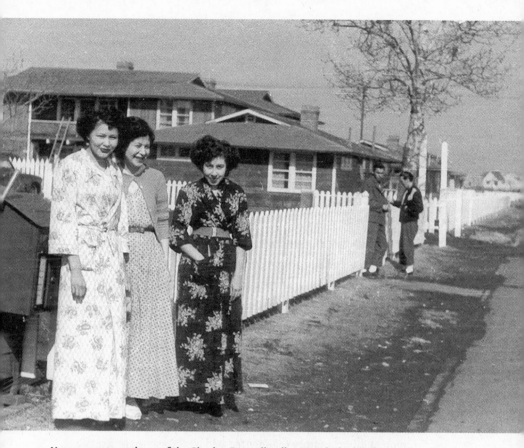

Young women patients of the Charles Camsell Indian Hospital take pleasure in fresh air by taking a stroll outside the hospital. Patients could venture outdoors with their doctor's permission, depending upon what routine they were assigned. Routines Three and Four allowed patients to be up from bed rest and walk on their own. [PAA 91.383.87]

Besides attending to their medical duties, nurses stayed busy maintaining their nursing stations. They might chop wood, paint, or even tend a garden to supply themselves with fresh vegetables in northern locations where produce was hard to come by. Their work was hands-on and varied, and it was this variation and freedom that many nurses enjoyed.

In addition to the work of nurses, doctors and their assistants travelled regularly to remote Aboriginal communities. Systematically,

IHS conducted annual tuberculosis surveys. Teams of doctors and nurses were sent out annually, usually in the summer and often at the same time as treaty payment parties, to make chest X-rays of Aboriginal peoples and survey communities and school children in residential schools for tuberculosis and other communicable diseases. In 1952, for example, ten survey teams were sent out with portable X-ray machines and more than 60,000 chest X-rays were taken that year.[25]

The C.D. Howe, a government icebreaker working in eastern Arctic waters, also participated in tuberculosis surveys among Inuit communities. The icebreaker routinely brought nurses and doctors into communities and then transported sick patients out. On Canada's west coast, boats belonging to missionary societies did the same work, transporting IHS health care workers and patients alike between islands and inlets.

Treating TB in Hospital: "The Routine"

Immediately after the Second World War, Indian hospitals offered a standard treatment regime for tuberculosis that consisted, first and foremost, of mandatory regimented bed rest. Despite the use of life-saving antibiotics as they developed, bed rest remained a central part of the treatment program. All patients quickly came to know "The Routine," a progressive system employed in almost all hospitals. Young and old alike, patients were directed to rigorously follow one of four bed routines depending on their condition. Each routine progressed to the next, and as patients recovered, they were allowed increased time out of bed.

Routine One was the strictest, consisting of complete bed rest. Patients were allowed out of bed briefly once per month. Those in Routine Two were allowed out of bed three times a day for fifteen minutes, but only at set times. During the rest periods, reading and talking were generally discouraged, and nurses patrolled the wards to ensure compliance.[26]

Routines Three and Four were less strict, allowing patients increasing time out of bed and even out-of-doors or away from the hospital entirely. Only as drugs and treatment regimes associated with new medical knowledge improved did the routine system lessen its hold over the daily lives of tuberculosis patients within the Indian Hospital system.

In 1961, in an attempt to educate patients about how to handle hospitalization, IHS published a small cartoon booklet, *Stepping Stones to Health*. Charles Camsell Indian Hospital patients were told that the booklet was designed "to help you understand and follow the rules of the Charles Camsell Hospital while you are being treated here. The information and regulations were prepared for your own good and many of them are part of your treatment."[27]

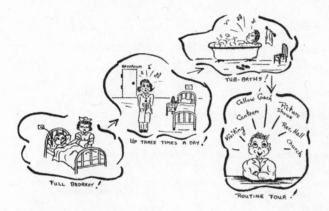

Stepping Stones to Health

An IHS guide for patients illustrating the routines for patients in hospital for tuberculosis at the Charles Camsell Indian Hospital.

Routine One

1. *Full bed rest.*

2. *Complete bed bath.*

3. *Your trips to the laboratory, X-ray, or to the dentist will be by wheelchair or by stretcher.*

4. *You may sit in a chair once a month while your bed is being thoroughly cleaned.*

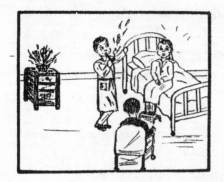 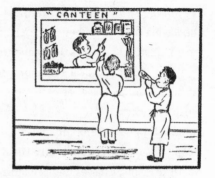

Images from *Stepping Stones to Health: Information for T.B. Patients.* This booklet demonstrated, in simple pictures and language, how new patients could expect to spend their time in the hospital. Posters and pamphlets circulated among patients in an effort to teach them the "rules" of the hospital and inspire them to better health practices.

Routine Two

1. *You may be up three times a day for fifteen minutes each time.*

2. *Bed bath—you may wash your own hands, face, and arms.*

3. *You may sit in a chair while your bed is being made each day.*

4. *Your trips to the laboratory, X-ray, and dentist will be by wheelchair.*

5. *Once a month only you may walk to church if your doctor thinks that your condition permits.*

6. *If you are allowed to visit on another ward, the visit will be made by wheelchair.*

Routine Three

1. *You may be up three times a day for half an hour each time.*

2. *You may have a tub bath on your bath day.*

3. *Your trips to the laboratory, X-ray, or dentist will be by wheel chair so that you will not have to stand while you wait.*

4. *You may walk to church on Sunday.*

5. *If you are allowed visiting privileges, you may walk for your visit.*

6. *With your doctor's permission, you may go out once each month for a drive.*

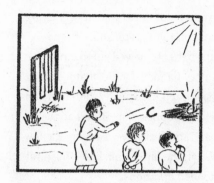

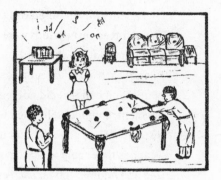

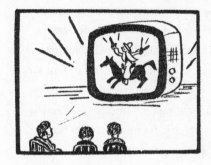

Routine Four

1. Except for rest periods, you may be up any time from 8:00 a.m. until 9:45 p.m.

2. You may be allowed to go to school in the classroom from 8:30–9:30 a.m., Monday to Friday, where classroom space is available.

3. You may walk to the Recreation Hall and the Canteen.

4. You may be up in your own room from 4:30 p.m. to 6:00 p.m. and from 7:30 p.m. to 9:45 p.m. Please be in bed at 9:45 p.m.

5. You may have a tub bath on bath day and oftener if tubs are available.

6. You may do your own shampoo.

7. You may walk to the laboratory, X-ray, or dentist.

8. You may go out once each month for a drive.

9. You will be given a red band to wear on your sleeve when you leave the ward on Routine Four privileges.[28]

Patients who endured this system of routines found it very trying. The enforced rest periods were difficult to tolerate, and, depending on the staff on the wards, many patients viewed enforcement of rules of each specific routine as heavy-handed. Unfortunately, many patients on bed rest did not feel sick enough to justify this strict confinement, compounding their feeling of oppression. Based on the testimonies of patients, humour and socializing were among the few weapons they could wield to chase off the blues from being hospitalized and regimented for such extended durations.

Beyond antibiotics and rest, surgeries were conducted where tuberculosis was advanced. These procedures included pneumothorax, or collapsing the lungs in order to rest the tissue, and/or orthopaedic surgeries to remove tuberculous bone.[29] Treatment for patients affected by tuberculosis in their bones (*tuberculosis osteomyelitis*) often meant stabilizing and securing their bodies—especially hips and spines—on specialized stretcher frames known as Stryker frames, or in half-body casts, for weeks and even months. Young children found this treatment especially difficult, not always understanding why they were immobilized for long periods.

The age, life experience, first language, and culture of each patient, coupled with the attitudes of nurses and caregivers, obviously played significant roles in the ability of those struck with tuberculosis to deal with their hospital experiences. Patients felt not only the physical pain and discomfort of a terrible disease, but they were also subjected to forced confinement, foreign environments, separation from community and family, confusing and sometimes bewildering Western medicine—all compounded by cultural and linguistic isolation.

NURSING AT THE CAMSELL

Marjorie Warke

Marjorie Warke and I met on a warm summer day in Comox at my
friend's house. My friend and I joined Marjorie at the large dining
room table, exchanging introductions and getting to know one
another. Marjorie assured us at first that she couldn't remember that
much, but as soon as she started talking, some of her memories
came back. To me, she was very concise and pragmatic with her recollections, not being one to embellish. She also had a few small black
and white photos, which she took out of her bag, featuring her as
a young student nurse at the Camsell with various patients. When
the interview seemed to have run its course, and we tired of talking,
I checked the tape recorder as a kind of break. Marjorie said with a
slight smile, "You got more out of me than I even remembered, now
that I hear it." We stopped there.

WELL, ACCORDING TO MY MOTHER, I was born to be a nurse. I was looking after her when she was expecting my brother and sister. When I was two and a half, I was trying to take care of her then, and it's been that way all my life. I was born in Vegreville, Alberta. Home of the giant pysanka. My dad was in the mountains. We moved to Edmonton when I was six months old. The only thing I ever wanted to be was a nurse. And one of my most favourite areas to work in, besides geriatrics, was pediatrics.

So, when I was in Edmonton in 1960 I was a nursing student at the Royal Alexandra Hospital. I was there from '59 to '62 and graduated as a Registered Nurse in 1962. As a student we all had to take a term through the TB hospitals. We didn't visit all the hospitals or sanatoria, but we did do our term at the Charles Camsell Indian Hospital. When I was there as a student, I worked mainly on the adult floor and a little bit in pediatrics over three months. Later I went back as a graduate and worked on the pediatrics floor, the non-TB floor, for a few months.

It was a fun time out there. We had a cottage on hospital grounds that we used as a residence. There were different students from different schools. Although we were still at school, being at the cottage was sort of like being on our own. Although we didn't really eat there we had snack food there. Mostly we took our meals at the Camsell cafeteria. The food was very good. When we were on night shifts, we really enjoyed it because sometimes they got roast moose and even Arctic char. And we could go into the kitchen and carve ourselves up a nice plate full of moose meat. The Camsell did provide some Native foods for the patients in the hospital. It was hoped that then the patients would feel comfortable. They were very well fed, the adults.

As a student, I worked on the second floor, which was a women's floor. That was really a lot of fun. We got to know the residents and we would go down with them to some of the different things that they attended, like social events and special occasions.

One of the interesting spots in the hospital was where they did recreational therapy. They did moccasin beadings and all kinds of Native craftwork, which was for sale to the public. I have a pair of

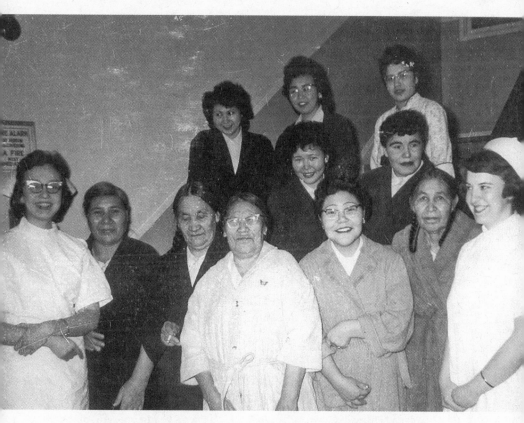

Marjorie Warke, RN (right) and patients in Charles Camsell Indian Hospital, Edmonton, 1960s. [Marjorie Warke, private collection]

moccasins and I have some soapstone carvings that they did. We were able to go in once a month, and what wasn't sold we had a chance to purchase. As student nurses we made a little pocket money so we were able to buy those crafts.

In the complex where the patients were housed things were of course not the same as their home surroundings. It was a hospital, a TB hospital, and so everything had to be very sanitary. The women's gowns changed daily, washing twice a day and such like. That was hard for people to get used to. I remember one young girl, she was getting ready to be discharged, and she had been in the hospital for four years. That's a long time. It was a complete change compared to what she came from, and I remember her saying, "When I go home," she said, "am I ever going to work hard with my people to try and change the way they live." And I remember the head nurse or the instructor, I can't remember which one, saying, "You know she's going back with high ideals, and it's going to be a real shock to her system. She's going to have a very difficult time to change what happens...It won't be long before she will be back to her same old ways." I thought that was so sad because she had such high ideals at that time and she would only be about eighteen or nineteen years old.

I also recall another patient, dear Lannie. I have a picture of her. She's ninety-four, a happy, good, old lady. The patients were very happy people. They didn't really complain. We had daily visits and played games, did the nursing care of course. That was good and interesting. It was a good time. It was a good time.

Was language a problem in the hospital? Not all the patients could speak English, so we pretty much had to use poor hand signals or a Pidgin English. By the time I'd been there most of them had been there a couple years so they had a smattering of English by then. I never really thought of it. I guess it was Pidgin English.

The Camsell was an old hospital and it had those old iron bed-steads. The walls were dull colours. It was not a bright cheerful place except for the lights, the white bedding, and the white upper walls. The gowns were either white or grey or that hospital green. It wasn't a lot of colour at all in there. And in pediatrics, the cribs were the old cribs. Like the ones in the pictures. It did need a lot of updating. But on the whole, the ladies wing that I worked on was a cheerful place, despite the dull colours and the white. They were happy. It was a good place to work and the feeling was cheerful. The hospital was not as modern as where I was trained; it needed quite a bit of updating.

When I was at the Camsell we were nursing students from the four different nursing schools. The regular staff were good. The young ones could get a bit ambitious, but then they were there a lot longer than we were so they developed ideas about what they were doing. And I think some of them—which is quite usual—had their

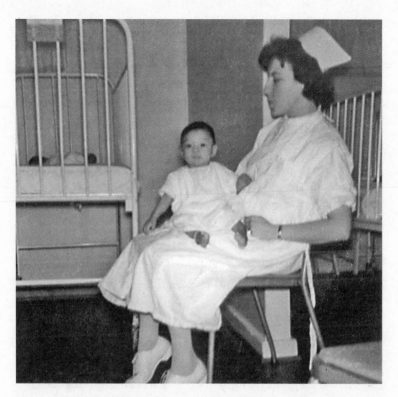

Marjorie Warke, RN, with young patient in the Charles Camsell Indian Hospital, 1960s. Ms. Warke recalls the old metal cribs and the rather drab atmosphere on the wards, but also the efforts of staff and patients alike to keep morale up. [Marjorie Warke, private collection]

pets. The patients that they really knew, people who were there for a long time. I don't think I saw any nurses or doctors being really disrespectful or mean—at least I don't remember that. Maybe I'm remembering through rose-coloured glasses, but if it had happened I think it would have stayed in my mind. I do remember one doctor I really had no use for. He was, well, I don't think he should have been there. I don't think he knew what he was talking about. He was on pediatrics on the non-TB floor. He was kind of rough and not patient with the kids and stuff like that. I didn't like him.

There were some Aboriginal people working in the Camsell when I was there. I'm sure they were on the cleaning staff and possibly in the kitchen. But I'm not too sure about the nursing staff, I think it may have been rare for Aboriginal people to be nurses.

I remember some of the children in Camsell. I just loved Emily. She was Aboriginal. She had a mass of black hair and violet eyes. And I just loved her. Every time I could, I was in there [on the ward] holding her and cuddling her. She died in my arms. She just died in my arms. She got sick. She was probably about one year old. I don't know what happened to the bodies of those who died in hospital. I don't know if they would ship their bodies home. She was there a couple of months, so I mean she had been with her parents. I just adored her.

When the young children arrived at the hospital, we would place them in the wards. One nurse would be responsible for about ten individuals, if it was busy. On the ward the children would be in those beds and they would be screaming. They screamed and they screamed and they screamed. And finally, I found out why. Aboriginal children were never left alone. They were passed from one person to another. They were carried in a papoose or on the hip. At the hospital they were dumped in a crib. It was so foreign to them. So, as soon as any of us had the spare time, we were picking them up and cuddling them and they settled right down. It helped them get over the shock. Non-Native children were very different. I worked on pediatric wards and the non-Native children did not cry like those at the Camsell. It was separation anxiety to the highest degree. If I remember right, what we tried to do on the pediatrics was try to keep the younger ones separated in different rooms than the older ones, so that, you know the ones that had been in there, and had been in there for a while were able to adapt and settle down. So to bring in the really crying babies was quite upsetting for them so we kept them separated.

When it came to visiting and having visitors come in to see their family members it was not like in a general hospital. There wasn't a lot of visiting at the Camsell because the families came from far away and didn't know or have transportation to come. There was very little visiting. Patients couldn't visit each other much inside the hospital either because of transference of diseases and stuff like that. TB is so contagious.

As a student nurse I did not give out any medications. I do remember putting hot packs on some patients, some wraps and such. Mostly we helped with hygiene, making beds, changing the beds, sorting laundry, bathing, and getting the meals to the patients. I do remember patients would sometimes horse around, like short-sheet the beds of their neighbours for fun.

One last thing I remember was one day working in the big unit, and we had the radio on. Then suddenly the news came on: John Kennedy had been shot. Oh! That hit everybody. That's when I was there, when he got shot.

OCCUPATIONAL THERAPY STUDENT, CHARLES CAMSELL INDIAN HOSPITAL, 1966

Truus van Royen

I remember as a very small child hearing about the Indian hospital in Edmonton from my mother, Truus van Royen. She always shares her recollections of the Camsell with intensity. For her, it was a cultural crossroads, a place that made a deep impression on her as a new immigrant who was keenly aware of cultural differences. Rather than interview her, I asked her to write her own memories.

WE CAME TO EDMONTON, ALBERTA, in 1964 from Holland. My husband started working in the oil fields right away, leaving me at home with two small children. Because I realized we should be independent from the ups and downs of the oil economy, I needed to work. I worked in Holland in health care but knew a Canadian education was necessary if I was going to be similarly employed here, so I applied as a mature student to the University of Alberta in the Rehabilitation Medicine program. That is how I ended up working at the Camsell.

It took time to get used to a new country, a new language, and the Canadian hospital culture was very different from anything I had experienced back home. I had a working knowledge of several Western European languages, which helped, and I made a serious attempt to learn a few Russian words from the Ukrainian patients. There were many patients, nurses, and hospital workers who had been immigrants at one time, as well as homesteaders who came to Edmonton from the North. The new immigrant workers were often a comfort to me. We understood each other's difficulties, regardless of our language, which could be a considerable barrier. I had difficulty understanding people at times, and they me!

The North had started to cast a spell on me. When I'd go to the airport to pick up my husband returning from the northern oil fields, the huge packs wrapped in canvas coming through the baggage chute had a mysterious appeal. Passengers dressed in long bison coats, or in parkas with fur trims, and some in clothes smelling of diesel oil disembarked from the plane. I was very curious about their lives.

Once, he brought little moccasins trimmed with soft squirrel fir for the children, and a pair of mukluks for me, beaded and tasselled. He said they were made by a woman in a local coffee shop in Indian River. I had never seen footwear like that, nor such intricate beadwork, and I wished I knew more about the country "up there."

Following my training, I had to make a choice of where my practicum would take me, and Edmonton's "hospital for the North"—the Charles Camsell—was at the top of my list. It was a sanatorium for long-term care of patients with TB. Many of these were from the northern parts of Canada.

On a Wednesday afternoon in the fall of 1966 I took the bus across the river to the yellow brick institution. It was not really inviting—rough grass in the front, a large entrance hall, long silent hallways with the usual drab grey and green painted walls decorated with yellowing photographs of Edmonton's early days.

I remember the sound of my footsteps when I walked along those long corridors from ward to ward. Wards contained four, white, metal-frame beds, with a night table each, and four metal lockers for clothes. The beige curtains between the beds and the mint-green painted walls come to mind when I think of the rooms. It was home for the patients. Some of them stayed for years before returning to the North. Many of them were quite mobile and walked around the hospital to the activity room and physio room, but some had to stay in bed, looking at those walls. I remember a feeling of total isolation, just looking at the person in bed, but relieved at the same time when I saw patients visiting and bringing drinks to each other and laughing together.

Sometimes I carried trays to people, who needed extra attention to eat at mealtime. I saw the look in their eyes when the white toast and the porridge appeared. I could not help but think of seal meat and hot tea from a metal mug I had read about in travel logs from the early explorers.

As an occupational therapy intern I wore a green skirt, a white blouse, and a starched cap, as well as sensible shoes. The uniform was not provided to us and it took me some time to save up for this outfit. I felt conspicuously "staff" wearing it, but started to feel more comfortable when I discovered that the clothes did not matter so much when we worked on crafts with the patients. Activities were our therapy, and I liked working with my hands.

I have one very vivid memory of my time at the Camsell Indian Hospital. On one of my first days I noticed the gift shop at the main entrance. The items for sale had tags explaining how they were made by patients and sold for the benefit of the hospital auxiliary. To my surprise I saw the same moccasins I had at home. I remember I held a pair of small moccasins in my hand to study the sewing and an old woman in a flowered dress and moccasins, came up to me and nodded. Her eyes almost disappeared in wrinkles when she smiled. I started talking about the fine quality of the sewing and the nice smell of the leather but soon realized she couldn't understand me. She kept smiling, though, and gestured with her hand to follow her.

I glanced around for the therapist, but I was early so I would not be missed yet, so I followed her to her ward.

In her room there were the usual four beds, the four metal lockers in one corner, the beige curtains, and that institutional green paint. Hers was the bed closest to the door. She had all her sewing tools on the nightstand. She opened the door to her locker and obviously intended to show me the rest of her work. I was almost overwhelmed by a sweet and softly putrid smell creeping towards me. A huge pile of green oranges filled the bottom of her locker. She was of a short stature, so she pointed to the high shelf, indicating that I was to help her. I stood on my tiptoes and found the package of moccasins she wanted, and quickly pushed the door shut. I had the sense that no nurse or therapist should see this green pile of fruit.

She pointed to my own feet and showed me some of her work, moving her hands in a way as if she was measuring me. No tape measure or hands touched me, she only used her eyes. I nodded that I would like a pair for myself. I still have them, a treasure from "up there" made by someone with whom I could not talk, but whose work I admired.

During practicum, the head therapist told us that most of the male patients wanted to do stone carving, but for many it was forbidden because of the dust and the fact that their lungs were compromised by tuberculosis scars.

I was familiar with TB because in Europe there had been a campaign with vaccinations and health measures and a lot of publicity after the war. As a child I was vaccinated with the BCG vaccine. It took me some time to really understand how TB had affected these patients. This was a different situation; the infection had been silent and misunderstood. The cure was very hard on the people because they were caught in a system to help them get healthy, but which put them in isolation far away from their families and everything they had ever known. The lack of communication due to language I felt was a big problem.

I think I remember that older lady and the moccasins so well because even though we couldn't talk, we did communicate somehow, and it was a powerful feeling for me because language was an issue for me, too. I do not remember paying for those moccasins. That still haunts me. I did not even know her name.

WORKING IN OCCUPATIONAL THERAPY
AT THE CAMSELL
Rae Dong

I met Rae Dong at the General Hospital in Calgary, many years ago, when I was a high-school student working as a "candy striper"—a volunteer helper on the various wards. Only recently did she recall her experience as a summer student at the Charles Camsell Indian Hospital in Edmonton. I told her of my research, and she immediately offered to share some memories of her time there. She made sure the story was just the way she remembered. Like others who worked and visited at the Camsell, Rae Dong also expresses that home-like feeling that seemed to exist in the hospital, even though it was an institution.

～～～～～～～～～～～

MY WORK AT THE CHARLES CAMSELL Indian Hospital was in 1963—a summer job for me between my university years. As an occupational therapy undergraduate in the University of Alberta program, I remember clearly how, on my first afternoon at work, the hospital administrator came to see me in the OT department, saying how glad he was that I could apply my skills to the department even though I would only be there for the summer months.

That kind of welcome was certainly rare and unexpected, particularly for an undergraduate filling a summer position. His enthusiasm combined with my youth and inexperience did initially threaten the existing staff as I was their "boss" and they were the aides. This "threat" was short-lived as we quickly learned to appreciate one another's abilities.

These skilled workers had kept that department alive over the years when no occupational therapist was available. They not only taught the skills of knitting, embroidery, beading and sewing of mukluks, mitts, and parkas to the female patients but also guided the male patients with the soapstone carving and small woodworking projects. Crafts were so important for the patients who were hospitalized for a lengthy stay as they recuperated from TB.

There was a camaraderie not only among the staff but also among the patients. They would help each other so that their end product was a successful endeavour. These items were sold through the OT department, and the individual was reimbursed for his or her work.

I could not speak any of the Native languages spoken by the patients, but we smiled a lot at each other and were very expressive with our body language and gestures. It was interesting to me that I felt comfortable in the knowledge we did understand each other.

I also clearly remember on first entering the building the warm home-like atmosphere which greeted you, not at all like an institution. The staff in our department ate together. We brought our lunches and we were like a little family. Few hospitals feel like that.

The majority of the patients were restricted to their ward and/or to their beds. Frequently we would take our lunch and join them at mealtimes to share the time with them. Much laughter occurred particularly when they saw some of the strange leftovers we would pack for our meals. The majority of the patients I worked with were adults over the age of thirty years. There were very few teenagers. But age did not matter.

I cannot remember a day going by when there was no laughter or happy music as we worked. It was such a rewarding experience for me, and I am glad the opportunity to work in such a climate was made available to me. It was a happy summer for me.

4

PATIENTS AND FAMILIES
Life In and Around the Indian Hospitals

I was afraid that I might be taken by the monkeys! The doctors were still taking X-rays of my lungs every day, and they had told me that I might have to have an operation. But one day I was told that my lungs were a lot better and I wouldn't need any operations at all. I was much healthier and they were going to send me home. I was very happy because I would be seeing my parents again. At the same time, I was a little sad to leave, now that I could go outside and was beginning to enjoy the south.
         —Simon Saimaiyuk, Inuit tubercular patient, 1965[1]

When I worked at the Camsell in the 1950s, that hospital was a gathering place for Indian people—almost like an Indian friendship centre!
         —Kathleen Steinhauer, First Nations RN[2]

IN WESTERN CANADA THE DAILY experiences of patients and their families with Indian hospitals varied tremendously. Many factors came into play, including the patient's condition and degree of separation from family and community. The location, size, structure, and staffing of the hospital also figured in the equation. Because so many patients were taken into care as children and subsequently endured lengthy hospital stays that sometimes lasted for years, these experiences fundamentally shaped their lives. For Canada's Aboriginal people, hospital life formed part of the fabric of collective memory, especially for those who came into direct contact with Indian Health Services.

Life in the Indian Hospitals

Perhaps the only way to understand daily life in the hospitals, from the perspective of those Aboriginal peoples who experienced it, is to encounter their stories, letters, family and hospital photos, and even the crafts and artwork patients produced both inside and outside the hospitals. Through their voices and views, we learn some meaningful truths about how the hospitals had an effect on First Nations, Métis, and Inuit individuals and their communities. The hospitals hosted complex social worlds where people of all kinds met and mingled— sometimes happily and sometimes not. For some, the experience of illness and treatment in an Indian hospital has so impacted their lives that it remains enduringly vivid to this day.

Accounts about life in the Indian hospitals come from patients, from family members, and from people with only indirect contact with the institutions. Stories from patients share common themes. First, they indicate that life in hospital was tedious. Recalling their childhood experiences in a hospital, many often related the difficulties from long periods of enforced rest. Children did not generally mix with adults, even if they had relatives in the same hospital. Many patients recalled how hard it was as a child to be required to stay still in bed for weeks or even months at a stretch.

Second, the stories characterize life in hospital as lonely. Patients missed their families, and, more often than not, because the hospitals were far away from their home communities and travel could involve significant expense, families could not visit their loved ones regularly, and some, not at all. On the other hand, many patients

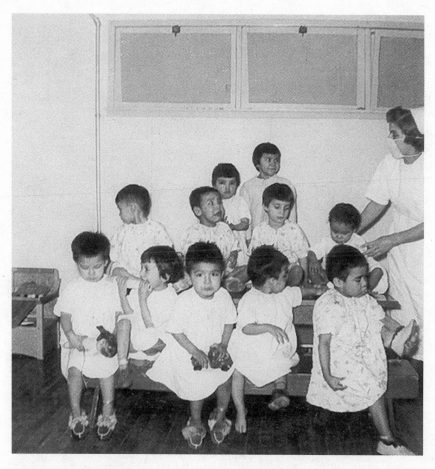

Toddlers pose for a group photograph at the Charles Camsell Indian Hospital, Edmonton, 1950s. Tuberculosis struck young and old alike. Very young children often found it difficult to adjust to the treatment regimes, which required them to rest and be still for long periods of time. [PAA 91.383.76]

had relatives as patients in the same hospital. Although having other family members with them might have provided a shared comfort, in most cases restrictive hospital regulations governing a patient's mobility made visiting a relative in the same institution difficult. Men's, women's, and children's wards often were located in separate hospital wings and little mingling was possible.[3] At the same time, some patients made deep friendships with other hospital patients.

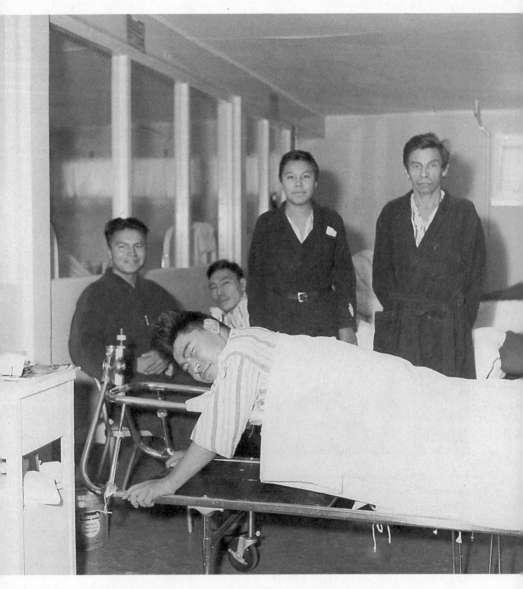

Patients in the men's ward, Charles Camsell Indian Hospital, 1950s.
[PAA 91.383.55]

Many accounts noted that upon discharge from the hospital, ex-patients found leaving those friends behind was particularly difficult.

Finally, some patients retain vivid memories of their hospital stay as both physically and emotionally hurtful. Language and cultural barriers between patients and caregivers made life difficult and confusing, if not fearful. Feelings of alienation from the hospital staff and separation from family and home could be intense. These emotions, coupled with the often-painful procedures associated with tuberculosis treatments, did much to emotionally scar both young and adult patients. At the same time, shared experiences provided camaraderie among patients that underscored trusted friendships and echoed Aboriginal principles of community within the hospital setting.

This story by Sara Saimaiyuk, an Inuit tubercular patient in the 1950s, encapsulates the range of feelings many patients experienced: "When I got to the hospital, all my clothes were taken away from me, maybe because I was more infected than the others. I never thought I was that sick. All this time there were no interpreters...At the time I was just a young girl and unmarried. I didn't want to go home because I got to like some Inuit in the hospital and I didn't want to leave them. I was in the hospital for three years."[4]

Though most ex-patients recalled the deep physical and emotional impact from their hospital stays, their memories are far from being totally negative. Many of their stories are characterized by humour, accounts of lighter moments with friends and staff, as well as examples of a stalwart determination to regain their health. Some chose to make the most of their recuperative years by taking advantage of the hospitals' educational and occupational programming. During treatment, many TB patients made new friends, shared pranks and jokes, and even learned new skills.

Patients frequently described music as an important and big part of hospital life.[5] Portable radios were popular bedside companions. Musical entertainers came to play for dances, or occasionally someone played piano on a ward. Recalling her years at the Camsell, Beatrice Calliou mentions how after her discharge she returned to work in the Ward VI kitchen, and "while on staff, I played the

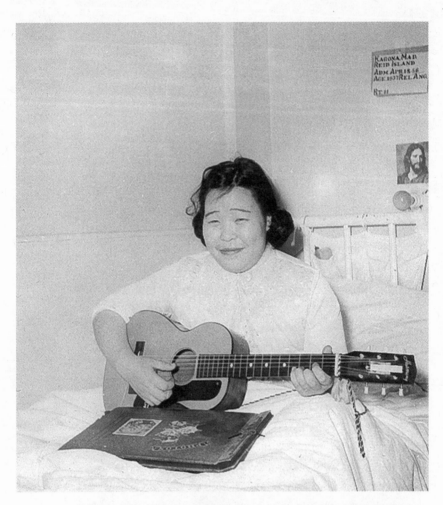

Ms. Kagona, a patient in the Charles Camsell Indian Hospital from Reid Island, NWT, strums her guitar while resting in bed. Patients became creative in finding ways to cope with hours of enforced bed rest. Making and keeping photo albums or playing and listening to music were popular activities. [PAA 91.383.85]

piano for a couple of dances at the hospital with Robert Gray on the guitar and Fred St. Germain on the fiddle."⁶ On the wards it was not uncommon for patients to play piano, mouth harp, or guitar. Gilbert Anderson, a Métis fiddler, recalled: "People sure felt comfortable at the Camsell. There was more acceptance there—it was a good setting. My brother Lawrence was an orderly there for a long time, between 1951 and the 1970s. He played the fiddle at the socials that happened on holidays and weekends. People really enjoyed the dances and the fun."[7]

In addition to enjoying music, TB patients in most hospitals appreciated the opportunity to engage in coordinated arts or crafts programs to relieve tedious treatment regimes. Drawing and painting were popular, as were knitting, crochet work, leatherwork, and other traditional crafts, such as beadwork and carving. In the Camsell, a handicraft program enlisted patients to produce traditional craft items to sell in the local gift shop. The department also hosted sewing and carving programs.[8] Through sales, patients were able to earn pocket money for themselves or buy new handicraft materials. Today, the Royal Alberta Museum in Edmonton houses a collection of arts and crafts made by Inuit and Indian patients at the Camsell for the hospital's "artifact collection," which it displayed in the hospital between 1946 and 1973.[9]

There were definite advantages to participating in art and therapy programs. In the Charles Camsell Hospital, for example, occupational therapy programs were relatively extensive, encouraging patients to "work" as a form of healing. Restrictions on patients' personal mobility usually prevented visiting between wards, but patients in the Occupational Therapy Department in the Camsell had privileges to visit other wards and hospital areas. This encouraged them to participate in various programs where they could see one another on a regular basis.[10] In the late 1960s, restrictive regulations began to change, making visiting easier.

School was an important diversion for some patients in the Indian hospitals. Many institutions offered at least some educational programs for its patients. Schoolwork helped pupils pass the time, and for some it was an opportunity to gain some new skills— especially in English—in preparation for their discharge. From the viewpoint of government officials, hospital schoolwork was also intended to have a "civilizing" effect on the Aboriginal patients, similar to the purpose of the Indian residential schools in the same

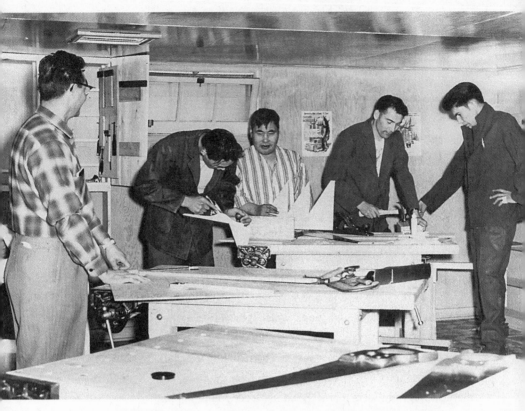

Male patients in the wood workshop, Charles Camsell Indian Hospital Rehabilitation Program, Edmonton, 1950s. Training patients in a skill or engaging in occupational therapy was integral to the healing program of TB patients. [PAA 91.383.97]

period.[11] For those well enough to visit a hospital classroom or who had enough energy to study from their beds, teachers offered books and exercises for students to keep up with their schoolwork. Teachers visited patients at their bedsides, or if the patients were allowed out of bed, teachers worked with small groups of students.

In the Nanaimo Indian Hospital, one or two teachers visited students and gave them bookwork to complete. In the larger Charles Camsell Indian Hospital, four full-time teachers and one part-time teacher augmented the medical staff, and classes were available to both children and adults from grades one to twelve.[12] Instruction was

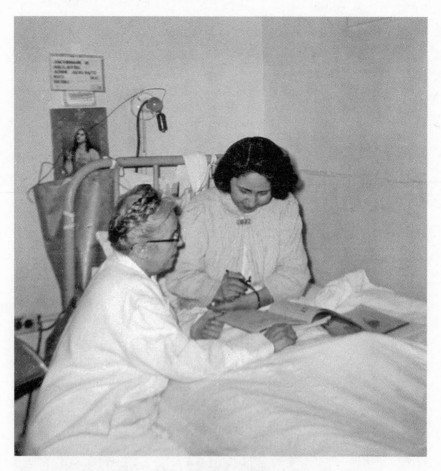

A patient at the Charles Camsell Indian Hospital, Edmonton, Betsy Jacobson receives tutoring from her teacher Mrs. Hanlon, while on bed rest, 1950s. School-aged patients were encouraged to continue their studies while receiving treatment in hospital. Only the larger hospitals offered patients this type of schooling. [PAA 91.383.87]

also offered in office skills, such as typing and shorthand. In 1952 at the Camsell, the school ran from September to April, and had 377 students. A small survey of students that year revealed that 75 per cent of those in the school program were working at an education level between grades one and three.

Visiting hours were an important time of day for patients; patients visited other patients, Aboriginal staff visited patients, and family

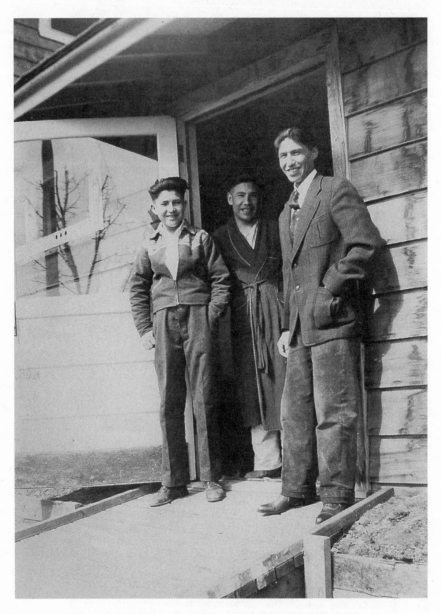

Patients and visitors at the Charles Camsell Indian Hospital, Edmonton, 1950s. It might have been difficult to tell the difference between some patients and visitors at the hospital, as patients in their latter stages of recovery were provided opportunities to participate in field trips into the city of Edmonton. [PAA 91.383.32B]

members spent time with their loved ones. Family and community members did not necessarily experience the full range of day-to-day hospital life. Those who could travel to the hospitals knew about patient boredom and loneliness, so they frequently brought books, craft materials, cameras, and even favourite snacks for sick relatives and friends. Patients well enough to walk could receive day passes to leave the hospital and visit friends and family off-site. This practice was more common in the later 1950s and into the 1960s. As Kathleen Steinhauer recalls of the Camsell, it was "almost like an Indian friendship centre!"[13]

Some patients dared to defy hospital rules and routines to sidestep visiting restrictions. Sometimes friends from outside tried to sneak into the hospital after hours. Ellen White remembered how her husband used a ladder to climb into a hospital window one evening to see a friend.[14] Doreen Callihoo, a patient at Camsell from 1946 to 1956, and then again from 1958 to 1959, recalled that during her second stay:

> I went back to my same old ways again, sneaking around and visiting my friends and breaking routine. By this time I was a little older and now I had boy friends. I remember I had a boy friend down on one of the men's wards. A couple of times I got dressed in my street clothes and went down to visit him during visiting hours. The staff on the men's ward didn't know me so nobody seemed to notice. I had quite a laugh over that.[15]

The *Camsell Arrow*

Another way that patients, families, and friends at the Camsell remained connected was through a publication called the *Camsell Arrow*, a newsletter edited by Camsell teachers and produced by the patients, workers, and staff. In May 1947 the first edition of the *Arrow* circulated to Camsell patients and staff. Patient contributions to the *Arrow* provided the readership inside and outside of the hospital a good idea of daily life on the various wards. Patients contributed jokes, poetry, short stories, or descriptions of hospital events. Whether the patients contributed all the details or whether the nurses for each ward helped write the stories, the entries for each newsletter reveal bits of patients' day-to-day experiences in the various hospital wards. Doctors and nurses also wrote short pieces for patients to instruct or guide them regarding their illness and hospital stay, as well as to feature community news. The *Arrow* also printed letters from former patients. As Dr. Matas, the hospital's first medical superintendent, explained in the inaugural issue, "We need a newspaper to tell one another what each one of us is doing."[16]

The July 1947 issue of the *Arrow* contained a letter written collectively by Ward III patients:

> We are happy to be back in Ward III again. While alterations were being completed we were moved to Ward IV. The ward is divided into four rooms, each with twelve beds. The walls are newly painted in pale blue and over each bed is a bed lamp....
>
> We enjoyed very much a car ride we had quite a while ago. We went to the South Side Park and took pictures. A week ago we had our second car ride of the season. We visited the Canada Dry Ginger Ale plant. We were shown through by the manager and all the details were explained to us. He gave us each a bottle of Ginger Ale to drink. On our way home we saw some of the department stores.
>
> Nellie Little Light had a nightmare the other night. She was chewing her shoe, dreaming that she was eating a piece of our native dried meat. When Maggie saw her, she understood, because she had heard Nellie wishing for dried meat.[17]

Demonstrating less enthusiasm, another patient from Ward III wrote: "I have been here a year and five months. My parents have never been to see me because we live too far away, about four hundred miles. I don't mind staying here but sometimes I do get lonesome. We go for car rides every Wednesday. We are very sorry that Margaret Burnstick and her little sister have been sick for some time. We hope they will be better soon."[18]

Like the patients, Camsell staff used the *Arrow* to advance their messages. Miss F.E. Taylor, director of nursing, used the *Arrow* to instruct patients on proper behaviour:

Please Remember!

What I am about to write concerns most particularly, I believe, the patients in the main building. It seems that every now and then someone upstairs decides it would be funny to throw a glass of water out of the window. I do not think that this idea is at all funny—it would be very embarrassing if some kind visitor who was coming to bring magazines, fancywork, etc. to you were the victim of your "water throwing."

PLEASE REMEMBER *in future not to throw* ANYTHING *out of the windows.*

I am happy to see that all of the women are now keeping their tables and chairs as tidy as Miss O'Brien's men on Wards IX and X keep theirs—this is really splendid.

PLEASE REMEMBER *to rest as much as you can every day—the nurses do not like having to keep on reminding you to take your rest, but they do want you to get better as soon as possible. So if we all work together "chasing the cure" you will be home that much sooner.*

Best wishes from the nurses.
F.E. Taylor[19]

Similarly, doctors advised patients on proper conduct for healing. In 1956 Dr. Matas wrote a reminder to patients in the *Arrow*: "It is very important for you to tell all your worries to the doctor or the nurses. The more we know about you, the more we can help you, so please let us know. A happy, cooperative patient is just as important as drugs and surgery in curing TB."[20]

For those patients whose tuberculosis went into remission or who were deemed "recovered," life changed after their discharge from the hospital. Some patients returned directly to their communities, travelling by air, rail, or bus; many kept in touch with their friends back at the hospital through letters to the *Camsell Arrow*. Frequently patients expressed affection and longing for fellow patients left behind. In 1950 Buddy Onespot, a newly discharged patient, wrote to his friends who were still patients in the Charles Camsell: "I hated to leave you all in dear old Tennessee (Ward 10C). Don't forget that I was once one of the gang...and somewhere in this world I hope that my trail will cross yours again."[21]

In many issues, former patients described their lives back home, their continued need for recuperative rest, how their communities still struggled with disease, and how families continued to cope with separation and the hospitalization of loved ones. The letters almost always included greetings to friends and family still in hospital, as well as to staff. The letters reflect optimism, gratitude, and a deep desire to remain connected with the hospital that had been their home for so many years:

From: David Tucktoo, Spence Bay, NWT
To: Mr. Dew, Principal, Education at Camsell Hospital

I am fine and in good plight always. Could you send me another Camsell Arrow? All personnel in here is fine. I am hunting and trapping this winter. I am doing well hunting. Our weather here—lots of storms this year. Good luck to you and God bless you. Remember me to all my friends and the staff at the Camsell.[22]

From: Delia Horseman, Lymburn, Alberta
To: Mrs. Heston, Teacher, Charles Camsell Hospital

Myself—I am doing fine, and Grandpa and the rest. Sometimes I go to a hockey game at Hythe—a little town just nine miles from here. I do enjoy watching hockey. Sometimes on a Saturday we go to a picture show. Maybe we will go this Saturday. Yes, I think I would be interested in doing some Correspondence Lessons. I do not know enough. Please let me know how much the Camsell Arrow and the Pictorial [Review] cost as I sure like to read them. I am staying alone right now taking care of the kids for my mom. She had to go to town to take one of my uncle's babies to the hospital. His wife is in the hospital so there was no one to take the baby. Just my mom....Hope I'll hear from you again as I like to get news from the Camsell once in a while. Say Hello to all my friends for me.[23]

From: Gabriel Sabourin, Fort Simpson, NWT
To: Camsell Hospital

Just a few line[s] to let you know that I am doing fine here at home. It sure is good to be home again. I was glad to see my friends and I'm alright now after a few days' rest. I was surprised to find my wife in the hospital when I arrived home. I believe she was very sick two weeks ago, but now she is doing fine and will be home again soon. I go to see her every day after taking my rest. I saw all my

NINTH ANNUAL

Pictorial Review

CHARLES CAMSELL
INDIAN HOSPITAL
AND
CANADIAN INDIANS AND ESKIMOS

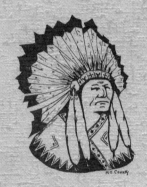

Cover of Charles Camsell Indian Hospital *Pictorial Review*, 1956. The *Pictorial Review* served as a "yearbook" for patients and staff at the hospital. Copies of the Review are today archived in the Edmonton Public Library and offer many insights into hospital life. [EPL OVERSIZE 362.11 PIC 1956]

friends in the hospital. They are doing fine. It is about ten minutes' walk to the hospital. It seemed a long way at first but now I make it without resting on the way. I guess you know that I had a baby girl at home. She was scared of me when she saw me at first. Now she is getting used to me. She's only 16 months old....
I went to the doctor last Monday for the rations I am supposed to get and he told me the Mission will have a job for me. I haven't gone to see about it yet.
I haven't had very much time to go anywhere yet because I rest before and after noon, besides I go visiting at the hospital every day since I came home. The doctor told me that I have to rest one year before I can work again. I'll try my best to do what they tell me....I'll start making wallets next week with the leather I bought. I have two customers already. I asked the doctor for leather and he said he'd ask the Indian agent to order some for me. I am glad that I will have something to do between rest periods. Please say "hello" to my friends in Ward 5C for me and all the boys in Ward 5 and 6 too. I'll write them later on.[24]

From: Ada Metchewas, Beaver Crossing
To: Mrs. Swindlehurst, Camsell Hospital

Dear Mrs. Swindlehurst,
I'd like to thank you for all the help you gave me. I wanted to see you before I left, but they discharged me quite suddenly. My parents didn't know I was coming back. I stopped by my uncle's place, which is not far from where the bus stops, they had a car there, so they drove me back here [home]. Mom and dad were sure surprised and happy to see me back. Now they make sure I don't work or overtired [sic] myself. It has been raining since the day after I came home. Although it rains it don't seem dreary anymore. I'm glad that I rejoined my parents, brothers and sisters. Will you please extent [sic] my thanks to Mr. Dosdall and Mr. Dew. This is all I could say for now. I will notify you if I receive my results. I am finishing my science here.
Sincerely,
Ada Metchewas[25]

From: Robert Laboucan, High Prairie, Alberta

I must begin my letter by again giving grateful thanks to everyone in our Camsell hospital. I shall always remember you all and how kind you were to me in many ways. If you don't mind you can make this known to all there and also say "hello" to them for me. I had to come to Miss Middleton's nursing station for a few days and then back to High Prairie staying with some Indians. I hurt myself some trying to work too hard, sawing and cutting wood. Likely I shall stay here all *summer, as I don't feel fit for any hard work. I'll be very glad to hear from you all. May our dear Lord bless and keep you all in His Perfect care.*[26]

The *Camsell Arrow* was an important bulletin for sharing issues and information among patients, their families and friends, and the hospital staff. It provided valuable insights into the challenges that patients faced, their hopes and aspirations, and their social world inside the hospital.

Aside from the *Arrow*, patients had another method of reaching out to friends and family from their hospital beds—radio broadcasts. It is unclear whether this opportunity was available in other western Canadian Indian hospitals, but at the Camsell, the Catholic priest set up a weekly radio program for patients to broadcast tapes of themselves singing or sending messages to home communities. The program was a great success, and according to former patients, family and friends eagerly waited by their radios to hear relatives' messages from the hospital. Even if the signal was weak, there was a sense of connection and keeping current with loved ones.[27] Patients in smaller hospitals probably did not have this opportunity and instead relied on mail or, later, telephone to communicate with their families.

Coping Strategies and Rehabilitation Programs

Separation and loneliness deeply affected long-term patients, their families, and their communities. When family members became institutionalized in the hospital system, some for many years, their families had to find ways to cope with their absence. Fathers were left with responsibilities to look after children, or mothers might be left without a means of income for their families. Some family members missed their sick relatives so much that they sought employment at the hospitals in order to be near them. Some husbands found work as orderlies or cleaners while wives worked in kitchens or as ward aides.

Through those fortunate enough to obtain hospital employment, the families and communities remained connected to loved ones who were patients.

After treatment, returning to "normal" daily life was not always easy. Life "on the outside" felt very different from a hospital with its familiar routines and varied but predictable activities. Some adult patients returned to their homes and picked up their lives as they had left them before illness struck. Others, especially those who had been admitted as youngsters, discovered that long absences and disrupted family structures seemingly made them virtual strangers in their own home communities. Still others chose not to return home and created new lives for themselves through rehabilitation programs designed to help them secure employment in urban centres.

Many ex-patients were too weak or otherwise disabled by their tuberculosis to return to their communities. Instead, they stayed near the hospital, taking work in the town or city where the hospitals were located. In 1956 the Department of Indian Affairs, aware of the plight of former TB patients, noted in a presentation at the Annual Meeting of the Canadian Tuberculosis Association that "...[Patients] must be given the chance to learn trades that their physical condition will allow them to undertake. It is further recognized that the kind of work they will be able to do is found for the most part in industrial centres....It is also essential to introduce them to life in the non-Indian community and help them to adjust to it."[28]

As the largest hospital in western Canada, the Camsell offered former patients a chance to enter into a structured rehabilitation program.[29] Created as a pilot in 1955, the program established housing for rehabilitation patients in a "boys home" and a "girls home" in Edmonton and offered education to upgrade their employability. The program provided training in trades like barbering, hairdressing, lab and X-ray work, office skills, carpentry, and cabinet making. Students could spend between six months to a year in the home until they had enough training to assume a job placement and take care of themselves in a private residence.[30]

If a hospital lacked a formal rehabilitation program, ex-patients sometimes stayed on to work in the hospital. For example, in the 1950s before her marriage, Marie Dick, a former patient in the Nanaimo and Coqualeetza Indian Hospitals, worked briefly as a ward aide in the Nanaimo Indian Hospital. Reports from authorities about other rehabilitation patients reveal a similar pattern of employment after treatment:

> Alvin Calf took the woodworking course with Jimmy before Christmas. Now he is employed on a full-time basis as a "cabinet" maker by a casket company in Edmonton. He seems to be adjusting well.
>
> Freddie Firth is working in the X-Ray Department of the Charles Camsell Indian Hospital.
>
> Sally Jackson is a successful rehabilitant and is now a stenographer in the office of an insurance company in Edmonton.
>
> Simon Jacko was one of the first to be placed in the rehabilitation home last fall. In November, he started a course in barbering. He is now employed in an Edmonton barbershop and is apparently liked and respected by the other barbers and by the customers.[31]

Outside of the organized rehabilitation programs, some ex-patients chose to return to the city after a stay in their rural home community. The April 1956 edition of the *Camsell Arrow* featured the story of David Koomiak:

> David, a 24-year-old Eskimo who lost both his legs below the knee six years ago, left the Charles Camsell Indian Hospital last spring to spend the year trapping in the Cambridge Bay area. He returned to the hospital last night in a flight with 12 other Eskimos from Cambridge Bay, and declared city comforts "look pretty good" after a year in the frozen north. Hospital officials will try to find him work in the city, Dr. Matthew Matas, medical superintendent said.
>
> Despite his artificial legs, he said he had little trouble making the week-long trips around his trapline during the winter. He broke one of his artificial limbs while at work on his traps but the RCMP provided parts with which to repair it. After six years in the city, however, the hardships of northern life seemed all the harder. "It's too hard," he said. "Work all the time." It was a hard winter too—"very cold," David said....

He spent four years in the Camsell hospital as a patient and worked two more years as an orderly before he became homesick for the north last March, and headed back to Cambridge Bay. Always a favourite with the hospital staff, he spent his first day renewing acquaintances with old friends. He hopes to stay in Edmonton for a while but may not be entirely through with the north yet. Cambridge Bay, on Victoria Island, does not hold much attraction for him now but, he confessed, some time in the future he might like to try the trapping around Spence Bay.[32]

IHS and Residential Schools

Life after a long hospital stay could be quite different for some Aboriginal youths. Following remission or recovery in hospital, some were sent on quite a different journey from other older patients who entered formal rehabilitation programs. It was not uncommon for the Indian hospitals to return school-aged children to residential schools—with or without parental knowledge or consent.

Indian hospitals and the residential schools were inextricably intertwined. Working in close relationship, the institutions sought to direct and control the lives of young Aboriginal peoples. Just as residential students found themselves transferred to Indian hospitals if school administrators believed they required medical attention, some teachers and administrators at the schools also endeavoured to create jobs for their Aboriginal students in the hospitals. Sometimes these jobs were positive experiences and gave students opportunities to work, other times, however, they served only in further distancing the children from their families and home communities. A good example of the connection between the schools and hospitals is illustrated by the recollections of Violet Clark. As a young woman graduated from the Alberni Indian Residential School, Clark found employment as a ward maid in the Nanaimo Indian Hospital through the efforts of her school principal. In her words,

There is a connection between the schools and the hospitals. I know my father tried not letting me work there, when I was 16, he thought I was too young to go out on my own. The school had made arrangements for the hospital and he wasn't sure we were looked after. So dad sent my brother down to pick me up. I was feeling so in the middle! The principal of the school told me it was going to be a good experience, and my dad didn't want me to. In the end it was my decision. So I went against my dad! [laughing] But I went home every summer for the last two weeks to visit. That made them feel better. Eventually he was glad that I did work there. I had an older sister that worked there for a little while, and then she transferred to Coqualeetza, and then from Coqualeetza she went to work in Vancouver, in a public hospital.[33]

In fact, Clark recalled several students from the Alberni Indian Residential School found some sort of employment in the hospital system.

In other instances, the connection between the residential schools and the hospitals was less constructive, from the perspective of the Aboriginal patients. Sainty Morris recalls in his story how he was transferred from the Nanaimo Indian Hospital to the now infamous Kuper Island Indian Residential School as a young boy. He received no warning of this move, and even his parents and extended family appear not to have been informed. He recalled,

One day the head nurse came to see me, and she told me I was going home. I was so happy! She said, "We are going to measure you for clothing and are ordering your clothes from Vancouver. Then you are going home." A few weeks later, the nurses came and brought me to change into my new clothes. I got a bath and changed clothes, and then I asked if I could visit my friends and relatives. I was allowed to visit, and they said, "We'll find you when the nurse is ready." Miss Fletcher finally showed up and we got into her car and started heading south, towards where my family lived.

We started going towards Chemainus [a town south of Nanaimo, on the way to Saanich]. I thought we were going to a store there, but when we got to the wharf, she told me to get out. I thought, "What is going on?" She told me, "You are going to Kuper Island Residential School." I told her, "No, they told me I was going home." That's when the nurse told me, "No, I've strict orders not to leave you until you get onto that boat." So I got onto the boat and they brought me there [to the residential school]. Everyone knew there was a new student coming, and as I was walking up the wharf I saw everyone watching me, whispering, "There he is."

This school was another awful place. They [the hospital staff] didn't tell my parents they were shipping me to Kuper Island! My parents didn't know where I was![34]

Michael Dick, in turn, found himself moved from residential school for treatment in hospital in Nanaimo. In his own words,

So, I can't recall the length of time I spent there, whether it was a year or two years, but it was long. Then one day I left. I was escorted out of that building by a Caucasian man—he took me on a ship. It was an overnight trip, I remember that, and when we got to our destination, I was surprised by the lights. I had never seen so many lights. I didn't know where I was, or what all these lights were! When we arrived he took me in a car, and we went up the hill, to buildings which were barracks. This was the Indian hospital.[35]

For Michael Dick, the move changed his life and he never fully returned to his home community of Kingcome Inlet on the northern northwest coast.

Undoubtedly, Morris's and Dick's stories are similar to events experienced by other young children who moved between the residential schools and the Indian hospitals. The connections between these federally controlled institutions were not always explicit, and often the only strands that remain of their cooperation are found in the memories of those who experienced that link. Despite the fact that the Department of Indian Affairs no longer administered Indian hospitals, the Department of National Health and Welfare was close enough to ensure that Aboriginal patients were never far Indian Affairs' control.

Weighing the social, cultural, economic, and emotional hardships versus the benefits generated as a result of the treatment system offered by IHS Indian hospitals is difficult. What is perhaps most important is that for many Aboriginal individuals, families, and communities, the experiences shaped by life in and around the Indian Hospital system's hospitals linger in collective memory. Although the historical fact of diseases, such as tuberculosis, influenza, and smallpox that devastated Aboriginal peoples, is indisputable, we are only beginning to understand the magnitude of the life-altering impacts of federally controlled Indian hospitals responding to crises in Aboriginal health. We can be sure that the complex and strict medical protocols in these government institutions left an indelible mark on the people and the cultures of Canada's First Nations, Métis, and Inuit.

A PATIENT'S MEMORY OF
NANAIMO INDIAN HOSPITAL

Laura Cranmer

Several years ago, my colleague Laura Cranmer discovered that I was researching the history of Canada's Indian Health Services. She told me that she was working on a play dealing with nurses and doctors and asked if I might have any interesting archival quotes or other information to help her with her play. It took me a year or two to realize that she and I were writing on the same topic: life in an Indian hospital.

One day, I worked up the nerve to ask if she would let me interview her. I wanted to hear her story. She considered my request carefully, and eventually she agreed. One day we both stayed late after work to record her words in my office. We laughed and joked around, swivelling around on our office chairs a bit to lighten the mood, but it was difficult for her to share her memories. I am so grateful that she did.

Laura's recollections emphasize how memories can be associated with powerful feelings, not merely events. These kinds of memories stay with us for a long time, and perhaps they say more than the memories of events.

Laura is currently working on a play, "Cold Needles," that deals with Aboriginal experiences of the Indian Hospital system (see page XLI for an excerpt from that work). She is an experienced creative writer and playwright, and today teaches First Nations Studies at Vancouver Island University.

This is Laura Cranmer's story.

~~~~~~~~~~~~~

I WAS BORN AND RAISED IN ALERT BAY in 1953 to my birth mother who was Haida, Pearl Weir. My father was David Cranmer. My parents met at St. Michael's Residential School in Alert Bay, where my mother grew up from a very young age. I don't really know precisely how old Pearl was. All I know is that she was barely out of toddlerhood when she was brought to the school, and that she stayed at the school until she left around the age of sixteen or seventeen. When she left school, she and my dad got together and I consider myself a sort of "love child" of that relationship since they got married in June and I was born in November. My paternal grandmother took over my care and the responsibilities of raising me from early infancy.

How is [it] that I was sent to the TB hospital? In some ways I'm guessing because I don't have anyone who, oddly enough, can verify which years I was at the hospital. I do have a photograph of myself just before I went to the hospital. It shows me all dressed up in a black and white gown with a little black cap holding a kindergarten certificate in front of my granny's fireplace. In the background of that photo, on the mantle, is a black and white photograph of my Auntie Glo, who graduated with her BA in anthropology in 1956. So my picture must have been taken in 1958, when I was five. I think I was admitted to the Nanaimo Indian Hospital sometime in 1958.

My granny, Sarah Martin, who was actually my great-grandmother, had tuberculosis, but I don't think my grandmother, Agnes

Cranmer, had it. I think I picked it up from my great-grandmother. I remember going down the stairs of my granny's house and being so weak that I would just fall down. I wasn't able to stand, I was so weak.

The next thing I remember was my dad taking me to Nanaimo. It was a memorable day because it was sunny and I [was] wearing a brand new blue dress. This was very unusual—to have a new dress was a real treat. Little did I know that I was being prepared! No one told me or explained to me where I was going or why we were in Nanaimo. When my dad finally got me to the hospital, I must have had a sense that once I went through the doors I wasn't coming out.

I remembered two orderlies coming to pack me, and I was struggling for all I was worth. As weak as I was, I fought against being put into the hospital! Only recently my dad and I were talking about this time in our lives. He said that when he was fishing he would walk from the harbour front up the hill to see me. I don't remember his visits.

I do remember the radiators because I burnt myself on them. They were big heavy things attached to the wall. I remembered the windows, and they would be really tall. I remembered being very fascinated by the TV.

Most of my memories have to do with body memories. I recall breaking a thermometer on the floor and being fascinated by the mercury, the little silver balls, and playing with them on the floor, and now I hear they are very poisonous! [laughs]

I also remember sitting in a bathtub and, I swear, they put ice in the water. I think I had measles or chicken pox, and I must have had a very high fever. I was hallucinating that steam was coming off the water, while really it must have been cold water and my fever was so high.

The other memory I have is of the constant X-rays. The technicians would make us stand against a big black plate attached to a kind of a metal column on which the plate could slide. I recall being pressed up against the cold black plate with my head tilted up over its metal edge and having to hold my breath until the picture was taken.

I remember other kids there, especially one of my cousins, Noley. We were the same age and on the same ward. I remember playing with her and watching the TV. I was fascinated with the TV and the cartoons. It was the first time I had seen this. I also recall being inconsolable because of a particular nurse being mean to me. When this nurse finished her shift, the next nurse came on and tried to soothe me, but it was to no avail. I just couldn't accept any comfort from anyone.

Of the daily hospital routines, I don't have too much memory. My memories are more about being hurt, or burnt on the radiator, or playing with the mercury. I remember being very ill and throwing up. When you're so small everything seems to be amplified or magnified in terms of importance. I remember covering the bed with my vomit and seeing that. I was just horrified. I thought, "What is happening to me? What am I doing?" I didn't know what made me [sick]. I think it might have been food poisoning. I didn't know what it was.

I was so impressionable. The feelings I remember were fear, uncertainty, and fear of not knowing what was going to happen next. I felt a profound loneliness, and at that age when you are so small, you miss the touch, that maternal, ongoing maternal love. I missed the cuddling and day-to-day things you expect when you are five years old.

I'm sure I had visitors. I recall getting a picture my granny must have sent me in the mail. It was of my Uncle Roy's wedding. I have this picture in front of me and I recall my response, which was "I don't know these people." My Uncle Roy married in December 1959, so it is through a series of milestones within my extended family that I can piece together my own timeline in the hospital. I really loved my Uncle Roy. When I first started kindergarten, I was told I would hang onto his back pocket and would walk along with him to school. Going to the hospital changed all that. The psychological, spiritual, familial break that occurred when I was moved into Nanaimo Indian Hospital so traumatized me that I repressed everything as a way to protect little Laura.

Today, I'm working on a play. The play has to do with imagining that particular space in a particular time in our history. The Indian hospital experience is one shared by many, many people, and we don't hear about it in popular culture. We hear a lot about residential schools, but as a social phenomenon the Indian hospitals had a profound impact on people's bodies and affected them mentally and spiritually. It touched them on all levels.

We don't hear too much of this, and I'm taking my experience, what I can remember, and magnifying and amplifying the details that would be provocative for a certain audience. What I can say about the current draft of the scenes I have is that it is quite slapstick. Although there is quite a lot of reference to death, there is also a surprising element of slapstick, even farce, and it is quite shocking to me.

Sometimes I think the entire experience was a mystery dream. When you are in the dream state, sometimes it feels so real, and it feels so real that you question whether it was real or not. You question whether or not it happened. What can you do when you have such an experience? This is my way of making sense of my history.

LIFE AS A PATIENT IN THE
CHARLES CAMSELL INDIAN HOSPITAL

Alma Desjarlais

The Charles Camsell Indian Hospital in Edmonton, Alberta, is one of
the few hospitals for which many records are still available. A large
and busy facility, the Camsell supported an active arts and crafts
program. It also published patient newsletters and yearbooks.
Many patients crafted, wrote, and photographed for these ventures,
resulting in a rich and interesting record of patient life within the
institution.

   Starting in 1991, oral histories were collected about the handicraft
program, and many former patients contributed interviews about
their experiences. In February 1992, Lisa Staples interviewed Alma
Desjarlais, from Frog Lake, Alberta, about her time in the Camsell
Hospital and about her involvement in the arts and crafts program
there.

   Alma Desjarlais's words remind us of the many hours patients
spent in bed, only able to read a little, or perhaps engage in some

handicraft. If they were allowed out of bed, many patients chose to spend their up and about times in the Occupational Therapy Department's craft area—one of the few places in the hospital where they were free to move about as they pleased.

Selling crafts through the hospital gift shop generated spending money for patients. Many patients spent their money at the hospital canteen, or used it to buy other necessities. Apparently, cigarettes were the most popular item sold at the canteen. Today, this interview can be found at the Provincial Archives of Alberta,[1] and it has been adapted here.

~~~~~~~~~~~~~~~~~~~~

Lisa Staples: What years were you in the hospital?
Alma Desjarlais: 1962 to '63.

LS: You were there for two years?
Alma Desjarlais: Fifteen months and one week to be exact. At the time no one got a pass, you just stayed there. I didn't go home for Christmas.

LS: What did you do to occupy yourself for fifteen months?
Alma Desjarlais: After I got better I did some upgrading and beadwork. I kept on from there.

LS: When you first got there you were on "routine one" where you had complete bed rest?
Alma Desjarlais: Yes, for six months.

LS: Were you able to do bead work?
Alma Desjarlais: I still did school work and read a lot but I couldn't get out of bed.

LS: How did the craft program work?

Alma Desjarlais: They supplied all the beads and that is where I learned to do my beadwork. Don't know how I learned. I remember the teacher...she is still around.

LS: Did you decide what you wanted to do; did they give you options? How did it work?
Alma Desjarlais: They asked you what you wanted to do. I tried different things, like knitting. I did the beadwork more. I watched my mother do the beadwork, but I didn't do it before going to the hospital.

LS: Did your mom do loom beadwork?
Alma Desjarlais: Yes, on the hide also.

LS: So you continued to do beadwork after leaving the hospital? Where did you get the patterns?
Alma Desjarlais: Yes. They gave us books and ordered from different areas and we picked out what we wanted to make. Sometimes there were special orders.

LS: Did you sell all of the work you made?
Alma Desjarlais: $1.25 for a necklace and they allowed you two necklaces a week. There was a limit on how many necklaces we were allowed to make. They had a payment plan: when you finished at the end of the week, whatever you finished you got paid for. The money was kept and I was able to save up to buy some new clothes.

LS: Do you know who were buying your necklaces? Did you ever have people order directly or did you sell through the gift shop?
Alma Desjarlais: Always through the gift shop.

LS: If you wanted access to your money, could you?
Alma Desjarlais: Yes.

LS: The wards you were staying in—were you with other Indian people from all over Alberta or in with Inuit people?

Alma Desjarlais: Yes, I was in with different people. The Inuit used to get dried meat and dried fish from up north and they would give us some. They had tattoos, especially the older ones.

LS: Did most of them speak English?

Alma Desjarlais: The younger ones did, and the older ones would get the younger ones to speak for them. The night before I came in, they had me sleep in the hallway. They used to get frozen fish once a week—like a Popsicle.

LS: Was it a nice atmosphere? What was it like in the hospital?

Alma Desjarlais: I guess it was nice. But it would have been better if I could walk around.

LS: So it was hardest to stay in bed and not do anything?

Alma Desjarlais: Yes, but once I was able to do school work and was walking around it was better than having bed rest. The funny thing is that I was in "routine two" for one year and then I was ready to go home. Patients got to go to a parade but I couldn't go to the parade. You were allowed to go home on "routine three."

LS: Did you have children when you went to the Camsell? Were you married?

Alma Desjarlais: No, but I would have had a hard time if I had any kids.

LS: Were there other people from your community in the hospital?

Alma Desjarlais: There was only one older lady. She went home before me; she didn't stay long.

LS: Did you have family come and visit you?

Alma Desjarlais: My brother was going to college and he would come and visit. My mom and dad used to come and visit me.

LS: What was it like for you when you went back home to Frog Lake, Alberta?

Alma Desjarlais: It was different. I don't know how to explain it. I used to go out and I couldn't walk around in the dark because I couldn't see. It affected my eyes and I even walked into a barrel one night because I couldn't see.

LS: How much school did you complete while you were in Camsell?

Alma Desjarlais: Grade nine. I came back and did upgrading. I don't remember the address of where I did my upgrading.

LS: Do you think that part of the reason you came back to Edmonton was because of staying at Camsell?

Alma Desjarlais: No, I don't think so. I did the rehabilitation option.

LS: I read that some patients were recommended to go to rehabilitation.

Alma Desjarlais: They taught us how to answer the phone and stuff like that. I went back home after grade ten.

LS: Do you remember other things?

Alma Desjarlais: There was a nurse from Sucker Creek Reserve at the hospital. I also remember meeting someone in White Court that I remembered. I met her at her parent's fiftieth anniversary.

LS: Did you have other family members staying at the Camsell?

Alma Desjarlais: I was the only one. I never got sick again after that. I would get X-rayed every year.

LS: How has the Camsell changed?

Alma Desjarlais: I was in the old building. Family could only visit for an hour and now they can visit much longer. There was no other sickness there except tuberculosis. I used to read under my pillows and cover my head and pretend I was sleeping. There were a lot of rules. We were told to rest.

LS: Do you think it was a good idea to have one hospital for Native people?

Alma Desjarlais: No, I don't think so. They should have had TB hospital for everyone. It's how I raised my kids. They go to white school and learn to get along better.

LS: Did you have just one teacher?

Alma Desjarlais: I had different teachers.

LS: When you were in "routine two," were you able to go to class-rooms or did you do your schoolwork in bed?

Alma Desjarlais: I could get up.

LS: Would you have any contact with the men in the hospital?

Alma Desjarlais: No.

LS: What about the children?

Alma Desjarlais: No.

LS: How about church?

Alma Desjarlais: Only the ones that were in "routine three" were able to go down to the chapel. I was Anglican. I got married in a Catholic church.

LS: There were only three floors in the old building. How many patients were on the same floor?

Alma Desjarlais: I hardly remember, maybe six to a room.

LS: Did you ever write in the *Camsell Arrow* [hospital newsletter]?

Alma Desjarlais: No and I didn't do the radio show either. There was a French radio station that we listened to. The old tapes have people singing, playing guitar, and speaking all different languages.

LS: Did you speak English when you were in the hospital?

Alma Desjarlais: Yes, and I spoke Cree with other people in the hospital.

I guess it was okay. It was easier for me than for some of the other people. The ones that had kids had a harder time staying there. My brother-in-law was in the hospital and he got a pass and didn't go back. He got medication; he went back and got the medication. The stuff that we drank was so bitter, in the cup. We had to drink it three times a day. But it must have helped.

I didn't have to go back after I left. They said I had a hole in my lungs. For a while they thought they had to operate on me, but they didn't. A lot of other people were operated on.

I get the impression that there were a lot of notices such as not pushing screens. We were on the second floor and used to talk with others below. "Routine two" I think went out for a while, and if you were in "routine three" you could get out more. I was only on "routine three" for two weeks and then I went home. I did not take medication when I went home.

A PATIENT AND A WORKER IN
BRITISH COLUMBIA INDIAN HOSPITALS
Marie Dick

The day I met Marie Dick I was visiting her home in order to interview her husband, Michael. Marie had been out shopping while Delores Louie (an Elder-in-Residence at Vancouver Island University where I teach) and I taped Michael telling us about his childhood and his training to become a licensed practical nurse.

I remember Marie coming home. Tired from shopping, she joined us in the living room of their small house. We introduced ourselves and quickly determined that she and Delores were connected through family. That led to a lot of laughter and questions. It also made our visit more relaxing. As we continued with our interview, Michael added that his wife was also quite knowledgeable about Indian hospitals. Marie humbly admitted that she knew a few things. It didn't take her long to remember details of her experiences. She was an unflinching storyteller, using plenty of emphatic hand gestures, and even laughing out loud several times during her tale.

Marie's story is short and powerful. It seems as if the memories about the staff are impossible for her to forget, so she started her story with those.

~~~~~~~~~~~~~~

THE HOSPITALS WERE JUST AS BAD as the residential schools.

The nurses in charge of the ward I was on called us and told us to be really quiet at the rest period, not to make a sound. "And you better have your table clean when I come on duty!" this one nurse said. I made sure I had nothing on it. Well, I had caught a cold and my nose was running and I put my Kleenex in the drawer. And my nose was running, and I had to get a Kleenex. I opened the drawer really slow. Just then she looked in the window of the door and she saw me. "So you're the one makin' all the noise!" she said. She came back with this ruler with metal on one side, and she made me turn my hands over and hit me with it. Just for getting a Kleenex! [laughs out loud] Never asked me what I wanted or what I needed. I bled. I swoll up. I could hardly hold my utensils for eating. I remember being wobbly.

Every morning the doctors came around, about three of them, like big shots with the head nurses beside them. Not one of them noticed my hands. And the ones that made my bed, not one of them asked me why my fingers were black and blue and cut. None of them! That is just one of my examples.

And then there were the two girls. There were two sisters across from me. One sister was by the window, just like me. I had a chair by my window, so I closed the window because a freezing cold wind was blowing in the room. That sister across from me didn't have a chair, so she rang the bell to call the nurse. And then the nurse came in, and the girl said, "Can you close the window, I'm freezing cold."

To our shock, the nurse said, "No! You're supposed to have fresh air!" The girl started to cry. And her sister got panicked, 'cause the girl was crying. So now they were both panicking. Even I was starting to panic! At eight years old!

"No!" said the nurse. So they kept crying. And the nurse said, "If you don't stop crying I'll fix you!" or something like that, and away she went. She came back with a belt, and she whipped both girls. For wanting the window closed.

From age eight to twelve I was in the Coqualeetza Indian Hospital. I went back to school at twelve, and I quit school at sixteen —you're allowed to quit at sixteen. So I was only in school for four years. I went from school and then when I was eighteen ended up sick again in the hospital in Nanaimo. Once I got out they asked me if I wanted to work as a ward aide. That's where I met Michael.

There were two ward aides for every ward. At Nanaimo there were seven wards: A, B, C, D, E, F, and G. The hospital employed two girls in each kitchen, as well. Every two wards shared one kitchen. We just served the food—we didn't work in the kitchen. We took out the trays and helped patients eat. In 1958 Michael and I got married, and he didn't want me to work there, so I stopped.

VISITING THE NANAIMO INDIAN HOSPITAL

Delores Louie

One day while at work at the university, I told Delores Louie about my research. She seemed very interested. When I asked her if she had ever been in the Nanaimo Indian Hospital as a patient, she replied, "No."

She followed my work, and later she told me that although she hadn't been in the hospital as a patient, many of her family had been. She joined me in my research work, came along on my interviews, and kindly advised me on my writing. She even began to find people for me to interview. After working together on this project for a few weeks, we arranged for her to come to my house and tape her recollections of the Nanaimo Indian Hospital. We drank tea, ate cookies, and then turned on the tape recorder.

The widespread existence of tuberculosis in Aboriginal communities impacted almost every aspect of those communities. Families were especially affected by the long-term convalescence of their loved ones in the Indian hospitals. Fathers, brothers, sisters, mothers, nieces, and nephews could be missed for years while their families struggled to carry on without them. Visiting the hospital was a challenge for many. Only those living nearby or with access to a vehicle could visit their relatives with any regularity. Being separated from family was something that even healthy relatives suffered.

～～～～～～～～～～～

I AM DELORES LOUIE—originally from Duncan, British Columbia. I now reside near Ladysmith, and the reserve I live at is called Shell Beach. Officially, we're called Chemainus First Nation. I've been married here for forty-eight years, and I have three children—two boys and one girl—as well as nine grandchildren, and three great-grandchildren.

Back in the 1950s I worked in the old peoples' home in Cobble Hill. I tried working with the Elders there, but I couldn't stand the treatment they were getting, so I ended up in the kitchen. I also worked at the Kuper Island Residential School. At the school I worked in the kitchen with the nun, Sister Veronica. She was the head cook. I enjoyed that.

I had a little camera back then. It was one of those little square cameras! I used to love taking pictures with it. Back in '59 or '60, my dad, Basil Alphonse, ended up in the TB hospital [Nanaimo Indian Hospital] for a number of years. I used to go see him. We were only allowed to go to the hospital on the weekends. Visiting was only allowed on a certain day.

We had an old vehicle, and I used to drive my mom to the hospital. If I think back on it now, it seems like we were there all afternoon, for visiting! I remember going into the building, especially the strong smell. Maybe it was what they used for the floors, eh? It used to smell like really strong sickness. When we went into the hospital for visiting, Mom and I would walk down the hall since my dad was far away at the other end. Hallways connected all of the wards.

The children's ward was another section, and I remember children crying all the time, as if no one ever bothered with them.

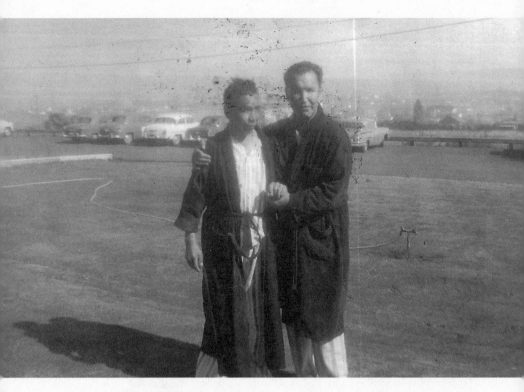

Basil Alphonse and friend, patients in the Nanaimo Indian Hospital parking lot, 1950s. The Nanaimo Indian Hospital was known to be quite hot indoors in summer, and patients were eager to get out into the fresh air if they could. [Delores Louie, private collection]

Dad said he got so tired of that. As visitors we passed through all the different little wards before we got to see Dad. The people there were all bedridden. All strangers. They weren't local people. I think they were from all different areas. They wouldn't allow Dad to get up at all, and from what I remember he was bedridden. Children weren't allowed as visitors in the wards, either. That could be hard on parents, the fact that children could only watch from a distance.

I don't know how others feel, but I always think of that smell in that building. I'd think, "There's that stench again!" To me it was very strong, and smelled like something burning or burnt. So this went on two years.

Then Dad must've gone for surgery, they took off three ribs, and then not too long after that, 1961, then they finally started releasing him. They started giving him weekends out, after which he'd go back in. So he was in that hospital for three years.

Did my family ever struggle while Dad was away!

My mother had two children she had to watch—my younger sister and myself. In order to keep us all fed and the household going she had to do a lot of knitting! [Knitting was an important source of income for many Coast Salish families.] Also, on weekends in the summertime we'd go potato picking. That was mainly how we made a living. But I think we mostly survived on her knitting. Of course, Molly and I were involved with the teasing of the wool, but my mother would just knit.

My dad was a farmer. He was a farmer all his life, working for different people, farmers. He helped with the plowing and all the other chores. He really gained weight while in the hospital. If you look at the pictures he didn't really look sick. But TB ended up taking his life. The three ribs he had removed for the treatment of his tuberculosis seemed to turn to cancer. So he passed on after a number of years.

It's strange. I don't ever remember the staff in the hospital. It seemed as if it was just the odd nurse we would see. I remember they were never around during visiting hours. I guess they would make themselves scarce—they were just never around. It was most likely they were in the coffee room!

My sister (she's actually my half-sister), my dad's daughter, she was in there already when Dad went in. Her name was Adeline. She was completely bedridden. I don't know how many years she was in the hospital, but she was there before my dad.

Again, what I remember most was that sickness smell, the smell of tuberculosis. I'd go visit Dad for a short while, and then I'd wander down to the other wing of the hospital and go see Adeline.

I don't remember bringing food, but I do remember bringing craft materials, because the patients did a lot of crafts, especially leatherwork. Dad used to make wallets, and Adeline started making wallets and picture frames, albums, purses. Patients also made little

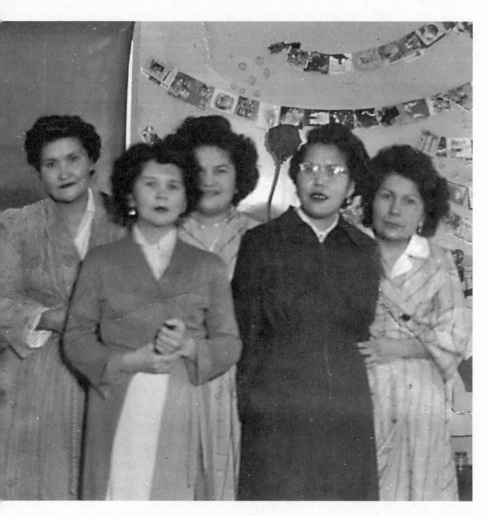

Women patients in Nanaimo Indian Hospital, 1950s. Patients could wear their own pyjamas and dressing gowns from home.
[Delores Louie, private collection]

baskets with neat little designs. They all sold things. It was worth buying even if it was costly for me!

In this photo [a group of women in dressing gowns] they are wearing their own clothes. They were allowed to wander around and be out of bed. My sister died of leukemia after they released her. She came out in 1963 or 1964, and one day she just collapsed.

My niece, Leona was her name, was only eight months old when she went into that hospital, and she was in there until she was eight years old. That was in the late 1950s. It seems that we weren't even allowed to see her until she was older.

Interestingly with Leona, when she came out her accent was like an Englishman. One nurse really took to her, and no one else could really look after her, and that nurse had an English accent. They didn't want to release Leona, but of course she had her own family to go to. Leona was the eldest. No other children in that family went to hospital, just Leona.

My brother Leo was only in the Nanaimo Indian Hospital for eight months. He didn't have TB, so it's strange that he ended up in there. He mentions that one nurse, Mrs. Langlois, just brought him in there to be checked and they kept him. He just had pleurisy. He walked out of the hospital. He got tired of it and just left one day. Walked out. He said he'd never return.

Once he was home he went on herb medicine [traditional medicine]. He got better in no time. His mom, our mom, made the medicine! His wife also knew how to make that medicine. Those herbs are really interesting. It was pine tree bark, and gosh, a few other ingredients. The medicine had three ingredients in it and it was made into a tea. He mentions that when he had three gallons, he drank that completely. The doctors checked him months after and there was nothing. He went back to logging! He was a logger.

That hospital, it seems like it just existed and that we just accepted it. We accepted what was happening to our people. It wasn't good or bad. My sister never ever complained about it. But when she did come out, she just said she just never ever wanted to go back. Same with Dad. He never ever wanted to go back in there either! Even my brother, today I tried questioning him, and he said he just never wanted to be there. I guess because they weren't allowed to walk and they couldn't visit who they wanted, or needed. It was most likely a very stressful regime in there. They were kept busy in there, but it was not good.

5

SNUWUYULTH

Local Indigenous Medicine[1]

 ~~~~~~~~~~~~~~~~~~~~~~~~~~~~~~~~~~~~~~~

IF WE LISTEN TO THE STORIES Aboriginal people share about their
experiences with the Indian Hospital system, we might be surprised.
Their stories counter the common perception that hospital medicine
and indigenous medicine were always at odds with one another. Did
hospital care stop or hinder local medicine? The stories contain the
answer as they reveal the value of examining the history of Western
medical institutions and practice using Aboriginal perspectives.

Although the Indian Health Services hospital in Nanaimo, BC,
provided modern scientific tuberculosis treatments to Aboriginal
patients, Coast Salish (Hul'qumi'num) notions of "medicine" were
also at work in this institution. Not always visible, indigenous
medicine was there, and health care workers in IHS facilities were
at times aware of, and even accommodated, this local indigenous
medicine. Community stories illustrate that rather than dichotomiz-
ing "traditional" and formal health care, notions of wellness, care,
and medicine were fluid within the Indian Hospital system, and that

patients and non-Aboriginal health care professionals like nurses and doctors negotiated that fluidity.

From the viewpoint of historian Mary-Ellen Kelm, Indian Health Services aimed to legitimize colonial relations and encourage the assimilation of Aboriginal peoples, this time at the level of Aboriginal bodies.[2] Laws and policies were devised to enforce the treatment of Aboriginal patients with Western formal medicines. Using the governing structures of Indian Affairs, including the Indian Residential Schools system, the federal government ensured Canada's Western formal medical system had access to Aboriginal patients, with or without the patients' consent.

Similarly another historian, Kathryn McPherson, identifies how, from 1945 to 1970, Indian Health Services and its staff of doctors and nurses continued to operate as a colonizing force in Aboriginal communities. From her perspective, IHS undermined traditional Aboriginal medical traditions, offered contradictory services in Aboriginal communities, and underfunded its system while maintaining relatively strict authoritarian control over its clients and their bodies, as a form of what she described as coercive "charity."[3]

Both writers point out that IHS—as a government institution—did little to recognize or work with Aboriginal knowledge associated with health care or healing.[4] Yet, McPherson suggests, at a local level, in the field and in practice, it is ironic that IHS nurses and health practitioners worked around IHS's coercive colonizing structures to provide Aboriginal peoples chances to assert their own definitions of health and care.[5]

Thus, local indigenous medical practices continued to co-exist with Western formal medicine despite the countervailing forces of federal Indian policy, law, and the actual biomedical treatments offered to Aboriginal peoples through Indian Health Services facilities and programs. But, specifically, we must ask, *how* did First Nations "medicines" and healing practices fare, and *how* did they operate in a context where Indian Health Services administrators and health care providers officially dismissed their value?

Based on my interviews with First Nations community members in the central Vancouver Island region, it appears that "Indian medicine" continued to be administered and shared at the same time and even in the same space as formal Western medical treatments offered by IHS between 1945 and the 1970s.[6] As such, "Indian medicine" constitutes a significant part of the rich and culturally diverse Canadian medical history. The use of local First Nations "medicine" within IHS's Nanaimo Indian Hospital in the postwar period provides a small glimpse into the nature of that co-existence, using Aboriginal perspectives.

A central theme conveyed in the oral histories that I collected is that "Indian medicines" moved fluidly in and out of the Indian hospital setting where Western formal medicine was also practiced. This indigenous medicine was sometimes highly visible in the hospital and at other times rested almost invisibly in the relationships between the carrier of the medicine and the recipient or patient. Sometimes IHS doctors encouraged the use of "Indian medicines," while other times they were seemingly unaware of their presence. The Indian hospitals offered spaces where medicine moved in and out, depending on availability of practitioners and on the needs of patients. As Kelm points out, "Aboriginal people did not relinquish their belief in their own medicine and its role in preserving their health."[7] Based on oral history, local First Nations medicines made their way into and operated within the very Western facilities created to subvert them.

Although Kelm describes how First Nations healing traditions continued despite the presence of Indian Health Services and their treatments, *how* local medicines were employed remains somewhat vague. Based on the interviews I collected, it appears that First Nations did bring their own treatments to the hospital in Nanaimo, whether or not they were invited to do so by physicians or nurses.

These "medicines" may indeed have been invisible at times; hospital staff may not even have realized that their visiting family members were offering local "medicines" to patients because the staff may not have recognized the activities of family as constituting the administration of "medicine." In this way, the bringing of food, the sharing of time and attention, and the administration of herbal remedies and special rituals went on in Nanaimo Indian Hospital without much notice.

Coast Salish "Medicine"

In the central Vancouver Island region, Hul'qumi'num-speaking peoples possess a deep and complex philosophy pertaining to the human body and how to best maintain an individual person's health and wellness. As part of this philosophy, myriad well-established cultural practices, both individual and communal, serve to enhance people's well-being by dealing with illness and sickness of all kinds. These practices build strength and support ongoing health. These activities might include, among other things: bathing, specific training exercises, eating particular foods, engaging in prayer and singing, and specific rituals. Herbal preparations and their application often form another element in treating illness and supporting good health.

Although generally many of the practices and preparations are commonly known and communally shared among members of the mid-island First Nations communities, some practices and treatments are kept within specific families, to be used only by those families or by special request. Some practices and preparations are deeply private and never shared, except in exceptional circumstances.

Taken together, these elements form the "medicine" upon which many First Nations peoples draw in times of challenge and illness. Generalizations about the nature and implementation of this "medicine" are difficult to make, given the sometimes confidential and often private way in which the "medicine" is shared and implemented. What is clear is that there exists a body of thought and practice that supports one another in offering humans a way to be a good person and to stay physically, mentally, and spiritually well.

Perhaps one of the more public aspects of this philosophy of maintaining good health is the body of wisdom known in the Hul'qumi'num language as *snuwuyulth*.[8] *Snuwuyulth* are the teachings offered by the Elders to those people who are willing listen and open to the teachings that offer guidelines or life lessons that convey the life skills necessary not only to be well but also to be a good person. *Snuwuyulth* is often offered through storytelling, from which listeners can draw needed information to help themselves. Shared both publicly and privately, the teachings are all-encompassing, addressing the mental, physical, and spiritual aspects of a person.

If a person is feeling unwell, family or community members offer *snuwuyulth* as a balm or a healing to that individual. In this way, *snuwuyulth* forms a type of "medicine" and is understood as such. These teachings assist a person to rebalance personal energies, body and mind. For example, some teachings deal with anger management or offer techniques concerning ways a person can deal with negative emotions. Other teachings emphasize how people should relate to one another to maintain healthy communities, such as including children in daily chores and knowing who one's family is in relation to the self. Some teachings deal with food, some with care of the body. If a person follows the *snuwuyulth* teachings, he or she is sure to have a strong mind, heart, and body and will benefit by being "well."

Coast Salish communities also have a long history of understanding the biomedical benefits of many plant components. In various families, there is traditional knowledge around what plants can be harvested, combined, and prepared to offer remedies for a range of illnesses. Ethnobotanists, such as Nancy Turner, have documented some of these remedies as part of ethnobotanical and traditional ecological knowledge studies.[9]

Likely these indigenous medical practices have been used for centuries. When Western medicine, a relatively new set of ideas, arrived with the Euro-Americans, some of these practices may not have been as apparent to the newcomers, but I have no doubt that First Nations "medicine" continued, often in concert with Western medicine. Indigenous medical practices continue to be exercised to this day, and in contemporary times as in the recent past, are frequently combined with formal Western medical treatments.

The Nanaimo Indian Hospital and Indigenous Medicine

The Nanaimo Indian Hospital was opened in 1945 as part of the Indian Health Services network of hospitals. It offered surgeries and drug treatments for tuberculosis, as well as other illnesses, although the vast majority of its patients were admitted for TB treatment and convalescence. Between 1945 and the 1970s, new antibiotic drug treatments emerged to address tuberculosis. Mandatory rest formed another important part of the tuberculosis treatment regime; fresh-air activity was encouraged for patients.

Patients and their family members who experienced the Nanaimo Indian Hospital in the 1950s and 1960s rarely speak publicly of their experiences within this federal facility. Yet a common theme emerges from some stories about Nanaimo Hospital—First Nations peoples continued to practice their own "medicines," both inside and outside the hospital, despite the availability of Western medicine.

The first person to speak to me about Coast Salish medical practices, and "medicines" was Ellen White, beloved Elder, author, and teacher of the Snuneymuxw First Nation. Mrs. White was trained as a young child by her grandmother in the preparation and use of certain herbal medicines, as well as in midwifery. Recognized today in her community as a powerful spiritual person and someone who has specific knowledge related to health and healing, Mrs. White spoke to me about her interaction with the Nanaimo Indian Hospital and the staff working there in the 1950s. This is a small excerpt of our conversation:

> My granny trained us in all the medical things by telling us story after story. Some stories are about childbirth. Or about behaving properly. Another story would be the power of words and how to cause problems for yourself. She also

talked to us about the dangers of using certain words when it's not right to do so, not proper. Words go with certain things and you are supposed to do it right.

The stories train us how to do things. We always say, "Remember that story?" when we are trying to do something. It's a lot like when you are being trained in the hospital to be a nurse. The stories taught us. We learned about kinds of medicines, how to stop bleeding with things like plantain, and a lot of other things.

I went up to the Nanaimo Indian Hospital now and then. I was called up there and did deliver a couple of babies. Some patients were sent out of the hospital. The hospital, I heard later, didn't want to have some of the women that were really badly affected with TB and refused them. It also didn't want some of those women to give birth. The doctor, Dr. Drysdale, would come in and later on, Dr. Schmidt....

I remember that hospital. I recall how one time [my husband] Doug carried a ladder up the hill, and how he used it to climb in one of the windows to visit a friend there. That's how he got inside! I was pregnant at the time and wanted to stay away. I didn't really like that place much and I got into trouble with one of the nurses so I had an excuse. I think she wanted me to stay away.

She said, "Its filthy stuff you're putting on the patients."[10]

As she mentioned during our conversation, one particular doctor, Dr. Schmidt, supported her activities. On the other hand, some nurses were less than appreciative of what she brought to the hospital in the form of knowledge or herbal remedies, and it was these individuals who eventually encouraged Mrs. White to stay away from the facility.

In another conversation, Mrs. White mentioned how she was invited to the hospital at times to help with "cleansings," a local First Nations ritual practice of sweeping out negative forces or energies from places thereby purifying a space or person. The hospital staff allowed her to come in and work through the ceremony for the benefit of the patients in the hospital. Undoubtedly, Mrs. White also shared stories containing the teachings with those she treated in hospital.

In these ways, Ellen White brought her traditions of healing into a Western medical facility that otherwise appeared separate from, and in ways ran counter to, local First Nations healing practices.

Much like Ellen White, Delores Louie from the Chemainus First Nation frequently visited the Nanaimo Indian Hospital in the 1960s.

Unlike Mrs. White, she wasn't invited by the staff to offer any specific treatments, but instead she came to the hospital every weekend to visit her father, brother, sister, and a niece who were all patients within the institution. Along with her mother and sisters, she visited these family members during the limited visiting hours. She shared valuable time with family despite the considerable distance of the hospital from her home on the reserve in Cowichan near Duncan, BC. In her words,

> Back in '59 or '60, when my dad, Basil Alphonse, ended up in the TB hospital... what I can't remember is who was first, my brother Leo Alphonse or Dad... anyway, Dad was in there for a number of years. I used to go see him. We were only allowed on the weekends. A certain day we had to be there. We had an old vehicle. I used to drive for Mom. Seems like we were there all afternoon, for visiting!

The importance of family and sharing time together is part of the Hul'qumi'num understanding of how to live well. When Mrs. Louie visited her relatives she brought them materials so they could work on crafts as they rested—crafts that they subsequently sold for pocket money. In visiting and bringing them work to do, Mrs. Louie offered her relations a chance to remain active and connected to the outside world. She was, indeed, helping her family in a way that was in keeping with her cultural values and teachings. Her family also assisted its sick members with herbal treatments, although they did not bring those to the hospital:

> My brother Leo was only in there for eight months. He didn't have TB, so it's strange that he ended up in there. He mentions that one nurse, Mrs. Langlois, just brought him in there to be checked and they kept him. He just had pleurisy. He walked out. He got tired of it and just left one day. Walked out. He said he'd never return.
> But he went on herb medicine [traditional medicine]. He got better in no time. His mom, our mom, made the medicine! And his wife. Those herbs are really interesting. It was pine tree bark, and gosh, a few other ingredients. Three ingredients in it. He mentions that when he had three gallons, he drank that completely. They checked him months after and there was nothing. He went back to logging! He was a logger.

Mrs. Louie's family used herbal medicines when the hospital treatment failed to meet their needs; they took care to look after the health problem themselves. The hospital was not criticized overtly, but her family perceived it as a place where people were not treated in a manner that might always help them.

> That hospital, it seems like it just existed and that we just accepted it. We accepted what was happening to our people. It wasn't good or bad. My sister never ever complained about it. But when she did come out she just said she just never ever wanted to go back. Same with Dad. He never ever wanted to go back in there! Even my brother, today, I tried questioning him and he just never wanted to be there. I guess because they weren't allowed to walk and they couldn't visit who they wanted or needed. It was most likely that stressful regime in there. They were kept busy in there, but it was not good.[11]

Significantly, Mrs. Louie emphasized the importance of visiting and staying busy. It is important to note that the hospital interfered with those important activities—activities that, in Coast Salish tradition, are taught as being good for a person's health and well-being.

Herbal medicine and ritual practices like cleansings were one form of indigenous medicine. Another was the normalization of relations through maintaining family and community connections through visiting and supporting traditional activities.

A third way in which local First Nations maintained and supported health was through gifts of food to patients in the institution. Officially, the Nanaimo Hospital provided meals for all patients, however, many family members brought their ailing hospitalized relatives preferred local foods to help them get better. From a First Nations perspective, the indigenous foods constituted another form of "medicine" or health care.

Violet Charlie, well-respected Elder of the Cowichan Tribes in Duncan, BC, spent four years at the Nanaimo Hospital as a tuberculosis patient. In conversation with me in May 2008, she mentioned how families brought food to their relations in hospital, especially the much prized "super-food"—oolichan (sometimes called "candlefish") and oolichan oil, colloquially called "grease."

LMD: *Someone would bring it in—a family member would bring it in?*
Violet Charlie: *Uh-huh. A family member would bring it—this grease.*

LMD: *And did they bring in fish and things like that for people?*
Violet Charlie: *Ya, they got dried fish, abalone—I never tried that—and they called it [oolichan] candlefish, tiny. I tried it and it's really rich. The nurses didn't object. Mind you, that was the four years I spent in there.*[12]

In this case, the Nanaimo Indian Hospital allowed family members to bring food in, although this was done at the discretion of the nursing staff and doctors of the facility.[13] The "grease" referred to by Mrs. Charlie was consumed by many of the north-central coast First Nations communities of BC. Rich in Vitamin A, it is a traditional food that many First Nations consider vital to their well-being.[14] In addition to being consumed as a food, oolichan oil can be used to treat skin conditions, such as psoriasis or inflammation, and even stomach ailments.[15]

In seemingly small ways that holistically treated physical, social, and spiritual illness, First Nations patients and their family members brought their cultural knowledge and understandings of health and wellness into an institution that otherwise did little to recognize indigenous "medicine" or cultural practices related to restoring and maintaining good health. The perception that these activities had a positive impact on the health and well-being of First Nations patients is evident in their stories.

Between 1945 and the 1970s, the Indian hospitals in Canada were authoritarian institutions, charged with the legal power to admit individuals suspected of illness, as well as to treat them, with or without patient consent. The medical system operating within the hospitals was hierarchical, with clear lines of command and obedience, beginning with doctors, down through nurses, and ending with the various support staff. Biophysical diagnoses and treatments were fundamental to this system, and the social or spiritual causes of illness were of lesser interest, as were indigenous cultural perspectives on health and healing.

In fact, Indian medicine was deemed to be virtually non-existent in this era. As late as 1974, academics believed that "with the near extinction of other forms of Native healing, the winter spirit ceremonial has become the only major non-Western therapy at the disposal of the Coast Salish Indians."[16] Ironically, it was within the Western medical establishment that First Nations brought their own techniques, generally with the consent of the medical staff. Apparently, Native healing was not extinct.

It seems ironic, from a contemporary perspective, that medical staff sought to isolate and treat Aboriginal peoples within a hospital setting rather than within their home communities (which often were viewed negatively as unhygienic and unhealthy), yet they still allowed significant elements of that community to "leak" into their own tightly controlled hospital setting. In this way, "Indian medicine" was highly fluid. Perhaps it was the humanitarian appeal of having family visit patients; or, perhaps staff simply lacked interest in, or insight into, what visitors were actually bringing into the facility.

A second irony also emerges from the stories about health care offered by the First Nations Elders that I interviewed. Although their collective experiences with the Nanaimo Indian Hospital were generally negative, they all shared their memories with a great deal of humour. The humorous recounting of their hospital experiences added to their sense of self-determination and resilience as they recalled situati

ons where indigenous medicines and ways were being tested. The success of local "medicines" in a person's life seemed to add to that person's sense of power and dignity and their ability to overcome difficult situations. Such tellings also underscore the significant power of the "medicines" themselves. As Florence James says, "The traditional teachings of my family will carry us through difficult times and it's wise to share them and care for one another. In that way, we receive a blessing and become stronger. No modern medicine heals, it is temporary for symptoms..."[17]

In the end, the treatments and activities related to health care that were operational within the Indian Hospital system were far more diverse than official or even anecdotal accounts of doctors and nurses within such a system might reveal or suggest. For this reason, when it comes to iconic institutions like health care, it is important to investigate the perceptions of Canada's minority populations, including the First Nations.

Canadian medical history is a rich field with many different perspectives and experiences, all of which deserve exploration and consideration. In this case, Coast Salish perspectives on health care reveal that, contrary to the perceptions of "outsiders," indigenous medical practices took many different forms, were highly portable, effective, and continue to be implemented even when members of that community were and are perceived to be lacking in the ability to deal adequately with illness.[18]

A CONVERSATION ABOUT
THE NANAIMO INDIAN HOSPITAL

Violet Charlie

Mrs. Violet Charlie is a respected Elder of the Cowichan Tribes on Vancouver Island. As a young mother she contracted tuberculosis and spent some time receiving treatment at both the Coqualeetza and the Nanaimo Indian Hospitals. Although she is in her eighties, she still lives at home and takes her daily walk up the mountain.

Delores Louie and I visited her at home on a sunny summer day to ask about her experiences as a patient. We arrived early, hoping to catch her before she left for her walk. Luckily she was home. As we came up the steps onto the porch of her house, I noticed her extensive collection of small wild plants, in various containers ready for transplant. She told me those were important traditional herbs, some with medicinal value. In the living room we settled into our conversation about the hospitals, her daughter listening from the kitchen while cooking.

Mrs. Charlie's recollections underscored the difficulty of being a young mother separated from her family and children during her many months of illness. Even after her recovery the challenge of adapting to life back at home, with all the responsibilities of looking after a family, was also hard. Tuberculosis, and how it was treated, affected people for a lifetime.

~~~~~~~~~~~~~~~~

Violet Charlie: Sometimes patients had their own foods, like grease and things like that.

Laurie Meijer Drees: Would someone bring it in, a family member?
Violet Charlie: Uh-huh. A family member would bring it—this grease.

LMD: And did they bring in fish and things like that, for people?
Violet Charlie: Yes, they got dried fish, abalone—I never tried that—and they called it candlefish, tiny. I tried it and it's really rich. The nurses didn't object. Mind you, that was the four years I spent in there. There were quite a few of us.

LMD: Were you in there with friends?
Violet Charlie: Not all of them. We became friends...

LMD: You were on a ward with all young women?
Violet Charlie: Yes. The ward was a barracks, divided into sections or cubicles. There was a wall and glass...there were four or six beds to one cubicle, wouldn't you say, Delores?
Delores Louie: Yes.
Violet Charlie: I had a corner. You would be so happy if you got the window side! So you could look outside! [laughs] It was very boring. Yes.

LMD: Did they do any activities with you?
Violet Charlie: Well, not until you're getting better. Then you can do craftwork. I never beaded before I went in for TB. I did do knitting

before I went in. When I was knitting the nurse brought me some wool.

LMD: After a while you were allowed up, to walk around?
Violet Charlie: I don't know, after maybe two years I was allowed to get up. To go to the washroom. Otherwise I couldn't get up.

LMD: Did they allow you to go out on little day trips?
Violet Charlie: When I was in Coqualeetza I was out for a couple of hours. Out with the bus. I was in Nanaimo first, and then for surgery I went to Coqualeetza. I had a lobectomy.
Delores Louie: They didn't take any ribs off, eh?
Violet Charlie: I wouldn't let them! [laughs] They were going to take five, and I said "No way!" Yes, you really get lopsided.
Delores Louie: I think Dad's was three ribs.
Violet Charlie: Did they take them out, too?
Delores Louie: Yes. His turned to cancer after.

LMD: Did they explain your treatments to you? Did they explain what they were doing?
Violet Charlie: Oh yes, they explained. I didn't want to come home after seeing the X-ray, and seeing the spots. I decided they should take it off. They explained that it might just come back.

LMD: So you stayed longer?
Violet Charlie: I had two lobes taken off. Which made it difficult to have surgeries after.

LMD: Was your family able to come and visit you?
Violet Charlie: Yes, they were. Those who were able to come.

LMD: I heard of some people trying to escape from the hospital.
Violet Charlie: Yes, I wanted to. Because my mother was very, very sick...and I couldn't even walk. I couldn't even walk to the end of my bed. I wanted to, but I couldn't.

Delores Louie: How did you find out you had TB?

Violet Charlie: My mother kept giving me Indian medicine. She knew there was something wrong with me. She kept changing it. Try it for one month and then change it again. But I started throwing up blood...and the doctor was watching me. It was terrible. I was afraid I would spread it to the children. I had to get away then.

Delores Louie: Was that Dr. Goodbrand?

Violet Charlie: Yes, that's right.

LMD: Was he at the hospital? Or here?

Violet Charlie: He was the Indian doctor here.

LMD: So who looked after your children?

Violet Charlie: My husband took care of them, and my late niece took care of them, and my mother took care of my baby.

LMD: That was a big worry for you, I'm sure.

Violet Charlie: I don't know how many days I cried. It is a lot of stress, all the way around. Having someone gone.

LMD: When you returned did you feel healthy again?

Violet Charlie: It's kind of difficult, after being...I don't know what the English word is...being told what to do every day. And all of a sudden I had to decide for myself, and it's different again.

REMEMBERING INDIAN HEALTH SERVICES AND TRADITIONAL MEDICINE ON THE SNUNEYMUXW RESERVE

Ellen White

Ellen Rice White (Kwulasulwut), a highly respected Elder of the Snuneymuxw First Nation in Nanaimo, British Columbia, was raised by her family on Rice Island, off the east coast of Vancouver Island. She married into the Snuneymuxw community at a young age. Trained in midwifery and other Coast Salish medical techniques by her Granny Rice, she has carried these traditions over the course of her lifetime.

Her memories of the Nanaimo Indian Hospital and its place in her community are wide-ranging and extensive. She recalled doctors and nurses, and how she and her husband sometimes visited family or friends receiving treatment there. She mentioned helpful people and others who were not. Her recollections of her work as a midwife on her own reserve represent a landscape against which all other stories about the hospital fit. Her story has many parts and pieces and reveals "health care" as many different things—doctors, nurses, herbs, and traditional techniques.

Her story demonstrates how local First Nations medical practices existed alongside the structures of formal Western medicine, which was available—but not always. She described how some doctors and nurses from the hospital were supportive—though others were not. The hospital was created for Aboriginal patients, but sometimes it did not seem to want them. Ellen White's stories remind us that what was consistently available were the teachings and medicines that belong to the territory of the Snuneymuxw people.

Mrs. White shared her story with me when I asked her to recall the Nanaimo Indian Hospital. Rather than speak strictly about the hospital, she chose this story, demonstrating the complexity of health care. Always a teacher, she told this story a few times and made sure I was not alone when I heard it. Finally, one day, we taped it.

~~~~~~~~~~~~~~

WHEN I FIRST CAME TO NANAIMO—and this is over sixty years ago—I already delivered some babies and was making medicine. My mother-in-law didn't want me to do that. I don't know how come people started to call me "witch." They asked me, "Are you a witch, the kind that heals people?" It hurt my feelings. We don't call it that. My brother-in-law started calling me "witchy." Because of that, I decided I was not going to do anything with medicine anymore.

One day, my mother-in-law came over and said that her niece was pregnant, and that the baby was due any moment. She told us her niece was very sick and in pain and had been in pain all day. I told her, "Remember, I said that I am not going to do that [midwifery] anymore, I'm sorry." I asked her to find the Indian [Health Services] doctor, but I guess they couldn't find him. So she said I had to come. I told her I wasn't going to come, and that I didn't like being called "witch." She went away and she must have been crying. This must have been during the day.

Later, my husband Doug came home, and as soon as he got home my mother-in-law came over again. I hadn't told Doug yet what had happened. His mother said, "I have come back and I have to beg.

My niece Mary is really bad. She passed out twice. Her grandmother doesn't want to look at her."

We talked for a while, and finally I agreed to go there and help her. It must've been coming close to the weekend, as Sunday we always went to church. I told my mother-in-law I would like to have some time after Sunday to talk to her children, to the others. We went to church. Anyways, she went away and I gathered the, my medicine stuff and walked up.

I got there with my bag with all the medicine stuff in there, including the little mushrooms in the bag, the feather, and my oil. I went inside the house and Mary was lying right there, her sister with her. I told her she would have to move, and Mary answered, "I can't move."

"Okay," I said, "I'm going to give you some of this medicine."

I think she didn't want this medicine, since she said, "Oh, I don't like that. Is it weed?" I didn't have much patience with her. I told her she either do what I said or I would leave.

Then she stopped resisting. "All right then," she said. With the help of her sister, I got Mary up and gave her a little of my medicine, the little mushrooms, and some warm water to drink. She'd been throwing up, her sister said. I gave her that to eat and drink, and made her get up and move around. Half an hour later she felt better and we got her washed up, we got hot water and scrubbed her up.

Her sister was laughing because she had never seen a body like that. It was because she had gotten into my bag. She'd gotten into my mushrooms when I wasn't looking and had eaten some. Meanwhile, I was working on Mary, kept rubbing her and could already feel it—just Indian medicine. Mary was much happier now. While the sister was in the other room, I took my bag of medicine and tied it to my waist so that sister wouldn't go through my bag looking for it and eating it.

We fixed the small little bed from the other room and put a chair in the end and a pillow. I made her walk, and she ate and felt a lot better. In the kitchen, I made her plantain juice, explaining how it kills bacteria. Then I put down newspaper.

The sister asked, "Newspaper? Why are you putting down newspaper?"

I told her, "I don't want to dirty everything." She really didn't understand.

She asked, "Dirty, you mean it's going to get dirty?"

"Sometimes," I said. Then I turned my attention back to Mary, the sister who is having a baby, and told her, "If you want to go, you go, you want to go number two." This really made her sister laugh—she was just so crazy, and she just got worse.

I put Mary on the bed and she felt a lot better. I put a towel and a little blanket on her. She was already going into labour because of the way we pushed her in the opening. The sister asked me did I put my hands in there? Well, I had to explain to her that we have to open it and ask the baby to come out. She just killed herself laughing and asked, "Why are you asking the baby to come out? The baby can't hear you." I had to be firm, to tell her the baby could hear us, and her, too. My gosh, I'd never been in a birth like that one before or since!

Every time she had the pain I talked to her. I told her I would put the feather in her mouth, and for her to make like she was going to puke. My gosh, it started to work really well. I gave her some more of the medicines, the plantain, and stuff like that. All of a sudden the baby came out.

We were already waiting for the afterbirth when someone knocked at the front door. We were at the front part of that old house. It was the doctor. Mary's sister opened the door and she said, "The Indian doctor is finally here!"

The doctor asked, "Is this where the birthing is?" I called in the doctor and let him know we were waiting for the afterbirth. I asked if he wanted to take over. He said, "No, you seem to be doing very good."

That sister, she just couldn't help herself. She started telling the doctor things like "You know what the feather is for? She wanted Mary to puke and the baby just jumped out!" she said. I made her hang on to Mary's arm, and Mary was telling her to shut up in Indian, but that sister, she just wouldn't.

That sister, she wouldn't leave the doctor alone. She got his attention, asking, "Do you know why Ellen put the newspaper under Mary?"

"I haven't the slightest," he said.

She said, "When the baby came out, he was able to read!"

The doctor was just killing himself laughing. "Why are you so happy?" he asked the sister. Well, she sure told him all about what she had done, saying, "I took some of that stuff that Ellen gave Mary. It's around Ellen's waist, and she wouldn't gave me anymore."

Boy, that got me. I had to remind her, "I didn't give you nothing," I said. "You took it."

After the afterbirth came, and we washed and collected all the stuff, the doctor stayed and asked a lot of questions. He asked, "Why did you open the afterbirth?"

I said, "I have to let the blood run in a bit." He asked a lot of questions and I didn't really answer some of them. It was really something else.

My granny trained us in all the medical things by telling us story after story. Some stories are about childbirth. Or about behaving properly. Another story would be the power of words and how to cause problems for yourself. She also talked to us about the dangers of using certain words when it's not right to do so, not proper. Words go with certain things, and you are supposed to do it right.

The stories train us how to do things. We always say, "Remember that story?" when we are trying to do something. It's a lot like when you are being trained in the hospital to be a nurse. The stories taught us. We learned about kinds of medicines, how to stop bleeding with things like plantain, and a lot of other things.

I went up to the Nanaimo Indian Hospital now and then. I was called up there and did deliver a couple of babies. Some patients were sent out of the hospital. The hospital, I heard later, didn't want to have some of the women that were really badly affected with TB and refused them. It also didn't want some of those women to give birth. The doctor, Dr. Drysdale, would come in, and later on, Dr. Schmidt. Dr. Schmidt used me a lot. He was always encouraging me and came down to the reserve. He encouraged some of us from the reserve to train as health aides.

I remember that hospital. I recall how one time Doug carried a ladder up the hill, and how he used it to climb in one of the windows to visit a friend there. That's how he got inside! I was pregnant at the time and wanted to stay away. I didn't really like that place much and I got into trouble with one of the nurses, so I had an excuse. I think she wanted me to stay away.

She said, "It's filthy stuff you're putting on the patients."

6

WORKING IN HEALTH CARE
Aboriginal Nurses and Caregivers[1]

Coqualeetza Indian Hospital, BC: Indian Ward Maids—There were seventeen
Indian ward maids on the staff at the time of my visit. The nursing staff and Dr.
Barclay are having considerable difficulty with these girls. It might be mentioned
that there is a military camp within two miles of the Hospital, and several recent
incidents would indicate that a strong and watchful hand must be kept on the
maids.
>   —Dr. W.L. Falconer, Assistant Superintendent
>   of Medical Services, 1942[2]

More attention should be given to training of native women in first aid and care
of the sick. A start was made in this matter at Aklavik and several native girls
were given instruction with this in view. It seems evident that such personnel
will require more preliminary education than has been given heretofore, longer
training, and some supervision in their community centres....Such a plan is likely
to fall short of its objective without more public health and social workers to
undertake a plan of health instruction in the various community centres.
>   —G.J. Wherrett, Northwest Territories
>   Health Survey, 1945[3]

No adequate mechanism exists that permits Indian people to have input into
health programs.
                                          —J. Kirkbride, Regional Director,
                                          Indian Health Services, 1973[4]

Lots of people died from infections and various epidemics in our reserve communities in Alberta when I was young. I thought, "I want to be a doctor—then I would
help." My Aunt Margaret inspired me. She was a public health nurse. She helped
me get started in nursing.
                                          —Kathleen Steinhauer,
                                          First Nations RN, 2004[5]

THE HISTORY OF IHS INVOLVEMENT in the training of Aboriginal
health care workers is a significant subject that has not received
much attention. Not only does this history provide insights into the
attitudes of the federal service toward the training of Aboriginal
people in health care fields, but it also forms the historical backdrop
to the contemporary devolution of health care to Aboriginal communities. Because of this, it stands to provide a baseline for evaluating
and gaining insight into contemporary Aboriginal-controlled health
services.

Looking into the powerful presence and influence of Indian hospitals in First Nations communities, it becomes clear that Aboriginal
peoples were more than merely patients. Aboriginal peoples in
western Canada participated actively in Western medicine as health
care workers, caregivers, and support staff within the formal health
care system. Between 1945 and the 1970s, significant numbers
of Aboriginal people worked, mostly unnoticed, within the many
facilities that eventually formed parts of Canada's public health
system—including Church-run hospitals and outposts, as well as
provincially supported hospitals and clinics. Some Aboriginal people
found work within the more segregated Indian Health Services,
assuming all kinds of roles within its numerous facilities, which
ranged from nursing stations to the Indian hospitals. Others worked
within hospitals and clinics outside the realm of IHS.

What roles did Aboriginal peoples play in formal Canadian health
care? More specifically, what roles did they hold within the federal

Indian Health Services system? The reality is that the line between work for Canada's separate Indian health care system and the public realm was blurred for many Aboriginal health care workers. In fact, they moved between the two systems as their needs required or as opportunity arose. Among these workers, many trained in Western medical practice through formal education in nursing schools and programs; others found their way into this workforce via piecemeal training offered by special, federally sponsored programs or other charitable initiatives.

Archival records are not rich sources of information for this recent history. Because the majority of Aboriginal peoples did not occupy professional positions within IHS or in public health care roles, their names were infrequently recorded, and they did not feature prominently in administrative correspondence. Furthermore, both IHS and public health care employment data generally fail to distinguish Native employees from others. Yet, here and there, records do reveal the presence of Aboriginal peoples in Canada's health care system and, more specifically, the IHS system.

Where typical historical record keeping fails to note Aboriginal health care workers, the oral histories, photographs, and autobiographies of Aboriginal people provide real insight into the roles that Aboriginal people played in formal health care after the Second World War. Combining information gained from these sources with what is available in the historic record, a picture emerges of Aboriginal people as active and dedicated players in health care provision. In the case of IHS, oral histories and archival sources corroborate the view that: "[S]tatus Indians and other Natives have been virtually 'ghettoized' within...the federal Public Service, in general. That is, they have been concentrated in the lowest level of the bureaucracy in menial jobs where their knowledge of, and sensitivity to, their people had no bearing on the actions of decision-makers."[6]

Assessments of "ghettoization" aside, it is more important for us to ask about the experience of Aboriginal health care workers. What type of work did Aboriginal peoples do and how were they trained? In western Canada, including the "western subarctic,"[7] Aboriginal people joined the ranks of health care workers through their own dedicated efforts, as a result of community support, and, at times, with the assistance of IHS itself.

Indian Health Services Hospital Staff

Between 1945 and the 1970s, the Indian Hospital system was staffed with both Aboriginal and non-Aboriginal people. The medical staff— physicians, surgeons, and nurses—and other rehabilitation staff, such as occupational and physical therapists, were mostly non-Aboriginal. Many of these health care professionals were ex-military because of the federal government's policy of hiring military veterans to federal posts after the Second World War.[8] In addition to former military personnel, the hospitals frequently employed "displaced persons" or immigrants from war-ravaged Europe. Although data is scarce and unreliable, the number of Aboriginal people employed by IHS in health service roles appears to have been low across Canada.

In spite of the fact that the Canadian government made only piecemeal efforts to train Aboriginal peoples as health care workers, First Nations people worked in various levels of health care professions, ranging from orderlies and practical nurses to registered nurses and community health aides. For decades, however, the government revealed a lack of commitment to devolving responsibility for the actual formal practice of health care to Aboriginal communities themselves, a situation that did not change until the 1980s, following pressure from Aboriginal communities.

Just as health care is now recognized as deeply rooted in culture, it is also a highly politicized activity. For most of its initial years, Indian Health Services operated in a "top-down" manner. Expertise was perceived to lie with the administrators, not those directly affected by and involved in the treatment of the sick and their families. The attitudes reflected in IHS were a product of the general integrationist attitudes toward Aboriginal peoples that permeated Canadian government and society between 1945 and the 1970s.

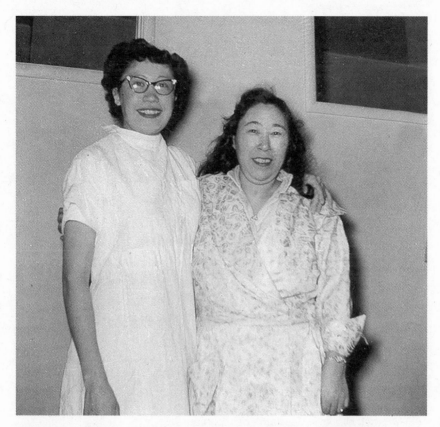

Staff and a patient share a smile, Charles Camsell Indian Hospital, Edmonton, 1950s. Aboriginal women and men worked in various capacities within the Indian Hospital system. Some were drawn to a professional career in health care based on their experiences in the hospital, becoming nursing aides, and even registered nurses in the federal Indian Hospitals. [PAA 91.383.79]

The creation of universal health care in Canada also worked against further federal commitment to involvement in Aboriginal health care. Despite that, Aboriginal peoples did play important roles in the IHS. Significantly, their work formed a nearly invisible backbone and significant interface with the Aboriginal patients in the system.

Given that specially created Indian Health Services facilities existed mostly in Canada's middle-north or subarctic regions, where provincial and territorial services were either thinly spread or not available, the question arises as to who staffed these facilities. Many of the hospitals and nursing stations were in or near Aboriginal communities. Not surprisingly, the nursing and medical staff in these facilities were almost exclusively non-Aboriginal. Support staff, on the other hand, were local and mostly Aboriginal.

Federally supported initiatives were important in drawing Aboriginal peoples into the formal health care system as labourers and health care workers. One early initiative emerged in the Northwest Territories in 1939, supported by a committee composed of the Northwest Territories Council, upper-level federal government representatives (including the director of the Indian Affairs branch, Dr. H.W. McGill), Indian Affairs medical officers, and Church leaders.

That year, a program was devised to train young Native girls as nursing aides in the various NWT mission hospitals. The course received official endorsement from the NWT Council in October 1941. The idea to create a Native nursing aide training program was not revolutionary. The Indian Affairs branch had already established the practice of employing Native people in its hospitals in service positions in the laundry and kitchen, and even on hospital wards as ward maids. Similarly, mission hospitals were training individuals under their care in various nursing techniques.

In fact, the plan to formalize a Native nursing aide training program in the NWT derived from a practice already in place at the Aklavik All Saints Anglican Hospital. In this particular case, the plan was thoroughly debated for over a year before being put into action, and it was warmly endorsed by all parties involved in the discussion as a way of encouraging employment for young Native women. It was also viewed as a means of improving community health should the trainees return to their homes. In his approval of this plan, Dr. Ross Miller, director of Medical Services for the Indian Affairs branch, stated:

> Concerning the scheme of training certain of the native girls while they are in the hospital…I think that this is a splendid scheme and the more such girls can be trained in the rudiments of nursing, the better the medical and health conditions should become in the districts to which they return after their training. These

girls could be known as experienced nurses rather than graduate nurses, because that is the term that is in general use throughout the country where they are of great assistance both to the surrounding inhabitants and to the visiting doctor, if any....Such girls, however, would be in a higher class than the home nursing group, because it would be advisable to train them more or less in operating room procedure and...partially trained dispenser of medicine.[9]

In turn, the Catholic Church endorsed the same scheme as a way to improve the lives of the Native trainees through assimilation into the dominant culture. Bishop Turquetil, OMI, explained, "There can be no question of considering their [Native girls'] training at the hospital as a chance to get married to white men, and so to give a better chance to these girls."[10] This same attitude was reflected by Dr. Miller, who believed that such training would be especially beneficial to "half-breed" girls, whom he believed to be "more intellectual" and who "would be infinitely better off as hospital ward maids than in returning to their native environment."[11] These initiatives were devised prior to the creation of IHS in 1945.

The Northwest Territories Council committee also endorsed the expenditure of government funds for Aboriginal students displaying exceptional talent and potential to complete a course leading to a registered nursing diploma. Such students were identified and moved to an institution where the higher education program was offered.[12]

The training program was officially launched in October 1941, and the mission hospitals in Aklavik, Fort Simpson, Fort Smith, and the Resolution Indian Residential School were enlisted to participate. The intention was to involve registered Indian, Inuit, and "half-breed" girls in the training, and the participating missions would assume responsibility together with the attendant physicians for overseeing the program. The Indian residential schools in the district, as well as the hospitals themselves, served as the recruiting grounds for students.[13]

In some respects, it is not surprising that the Northwest Territories was chosen as the location to launch such training. The region was relatively inaccessible, had an Aboriginal population suffering terribly from tuberculosis, and boasted one of the highest ratios of hospital beds per capita—four times that of British Columbia, which had the highest hospital bed complement of the provinces.[14]

The training, in this case, consisted of teaching students many of the skills taught to non-Aboriginal practical nurses or nursing assistants. The idea was to teach

> ...elements of dietary and plain cooking, take temperatures, do simple dressings, make up dressings, give enemas, properly make beds and give sponge or bed baths. They should also understand the use of simple cathartics and have some knowledge of the proper use of simple remedies which are used in every home, such as the application of mustard, the use of pneumonia jackets and they should also be taught the elements of hygiene with particular regard to preventing the spread of tuberculosis in the home and out at camps.[15]

Dr. H.W. McGill, himself a trained physician, added that students could be "taught to make beds, prepare hot-water bottles and assist in the preparation of meals for patients."[16] He believed that the aides would provide the minimum in nursing support. Young women were accepted into this training system as young as nine years old, as were adults. Earlier archival records of Aboriginal workers in Indian Affairs hospital facilities suggest that men and women worked as support staff, and some young women were trained within those facilities as "ward maids," employed in exchange for room, board, and fifteen dollars a month.[17]

Upon completion of the training, which lasted between eighteen and thirty-six months, students received an "unofficial" certificate signed by the medical officer in charge of their program. In December 1941, the first "graduates" were awarded certificates from the Fort Smith Hospital. Dr. J.A. Urquhart, the physician attending this Catholic mission hospital, proclaimed, "With this group, the experiment can be considered an unqualified success."[18] The Fort Smith Hospital was one of the larger facilities in the Northwest Territories, featuring a forty-three-bed capacity, as well as laboratory facilities second in size only to the Anglican hospital in Aklavik.[19]

This early program, characterized by a lack of solid federal support, low expectations, and an informal approach to training, could be viewed as the pattern for things to come in the field of Aboriginal health care training until the 1970s. Programs that followed within the IHS system were equally unsystematized and focused primarily on training aides and helpers, rather than promoting full certification of Native nurses, although some Native women were indeed successful in achieving registered nurse credentials.

One such example is Mrs. Muriel Innes, a young woman from Cowessess First Nation in Saskatchewan. Just after the Second World War and the death of her mother, her father took work at the Lac La Ronge fish processing plant in northern Saskatchewan and moved his daughter to the IHS nursing station. Mrs. Innes remained at the nursing station for two years, training with the IHS nurse stationed there. Her work ranged from preparing linens and bandages and sterilizing equipment to watching the outpost while the nurse was away. She recalled how the nurses at the La Ronge outpost had difficulty communicating with the Cree-speaking patients, and so the nursing station cook, a local woman, was used as a translator. Innes herself felt that the nurses with whom she worked were very dedicated, but she noted that, because their workload was heavy and time-consuming, these women never really integrated themselves into the local community. Following her work in La Ronge, Innes transferred to the IHS hospital at Prince Rupert to continue working as a nursing aide.[20]

It is unclear the extent to which IHS trained and hired nurses' aides in this informal manner. What is clear is that more formal practical nurse and nurses' aide training programs were spearheaded in IHS hospitals in the 1950s. In 1955, for example, the Coqualeetza Indian Hospital in British Columbia began running a formal practical nurse training program in affiliation with the Vancouver Vocational Institute. In this program, three trainees at a time were placed in the Coqualeetza Hospital for a two-month internship in order to gain experience in tuberculosis and pediatric nursing. Although non-Native women were involved in this training program, according to the IHS, "The course is becoming increasingly popular with Indian girls."[21]

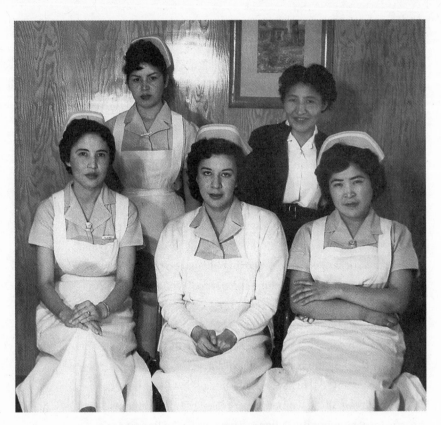

Aboriginal staff, Charles Camsell Indian Hospital, Edmonton, 1950s.
[PAA 91.383.237]

IHS assisted Aboriginal applicants with short-term jobs to "provide the initial experience and helping to put the Indian on an equal starting basis with the white girl."[22] A version of the practical nurse training program spearheaded in the Northwest Territories continued into the 1950s.

The pattern of employing Aboriginal workers as support staff continued throughout the 1950s and 1960s, despite a recognized shortage of nurses to work in IHS facilities. In 1952, the Hon. Paul Martin, the minister responsible for IHS, announced to Parliament: "We now have about 212 Indians in our service, although the number fluctuates. I fully agree...that we ought to make every endeavor to have as many of the native population as possible serve in this capacity. We have taken steps to get young girls to go into nursing training and have encouraged them in every way. Our success in that regard is not what I would like it to be."[23]

Despite his lament, few formalized training opportunities existed within IHS itself, and the service continued to rely on outside agencies to provide this education to First Nations people. The 1953–54 Indian Health Services annual reports mentioned Aboriginal staff for the first time. That year, 167 "Indians and Eskimos" were employed, and up to 250 worked on an hourly basis.

St. Ann's Hospital in Fort Smith, for example, offered training to Inuit, Indian, and non-Native "outsiders." A 1954 photograph published by Dr. Percy E. Moore was captioned: "A group of girls taking training as ward aides at St. Ann's Hospital, Fort Smith. In the front row are the first three Eskimo girls to take the course, and behind them are a German DP and three Indian girls. In addition to their practical work, they learn anatomy, physiology, ethics and hygiene."[24]

Similar ventures were initiated in other IHS hospitals. In general, the idea seems to have been that non-Native women were the most desirable to hire in these hospitals but that Native women could at least be introduced to nursing careers. Nursing in Aboriginal communities and in IHS hospitals was viewed as difficult, demanding, and highly specialized work, something that the Aboriginal population was perceived as not ready or able to take on in any professional capacity—with the exception of the occasional, unusually talented individual.

In the 1950s and 1960s, patients in IHS hospitals—often those undergoing long-term recoveries from tuberculosis—were also encouraged to seek employment in the hospital facilities, and it was common for former patients to work at the hospital once they recovered. Harriet Buffalo, a Camsell Hospital patient in 1948–49, returned to work in the hospital kitchens after her recovery. She recalled: "In 1953, I was employed at the hospital to work in the ward kitchens. I helped serve meals to the Eskimo and Indian patients, young and old. I appreciated the work and enjoyed it."[25] Although archival records documenting this trend are slim, the IHS directorate noted that, "as

soon as our patients are able, they engage in rehabilitation employment around the hospital. This is carried out on a selective basis."[26]

From photographs, documents, and oral histories related to the
Charles Camsell Indian Hospital, the Nanaimo Indian Hospital, and
the Coqualeetza Indian Hospital, it is evident that Aboriginal patients
were actively being trained and employed as orderlies, attendants,
X-ray and lab technicians, and nurses' aides. In-house training in
the Charles Camsell Hospital allowed patients and other Aboriginal
trainees to acquire their skills while "on the job," and classes were
held right in the hospital.

Generally, however, most training offered through federal effort
was for unskilled work. Aboriginal people filled many of the lower-
ranking, non-medical, support positions. In both the Nanaimo and
Camsell Hospitals, they worked in the kitchens, the laundry, in janitorial or minor technical positions, and on the wards as orderlies,
ward aides, and, in exceptional cases, as nurses.

In fact, in federal health care facilities, tuberculosis was seen as a
vehicle for training Aboriginal people. From the Saskatchewan region
in the IHS system, the view expressed was that "[w]hile one would
hope that Tuberculosis will eventually be eradicated, nevertheless the
disease has served as a medium for the academic training of a great
many Indians."[27]

This technical training was done through an informal
Rehabilitation Program launched in 1955 to train young people after
their TB went into remission but who were deemed too debilitated to
return home to their Native communities. These trainees were transferred out of the hospital to two local Edmonton homes where they
were taught basic skills that would allow them to work in a variety of
settings, including a hospital or nursing clinic, but not necessarily
back in their home communities. Discontinued in 1961, six years after

X-ray technicians at work. Aboriginal staff, Charles Camsell Indian Hospital,
Edmonton, 1950s. Patients were sometimes trained by hospital staff in
technician roles, and some found employment in this manner after their
rehabilitation. [PAA 91.383.413]

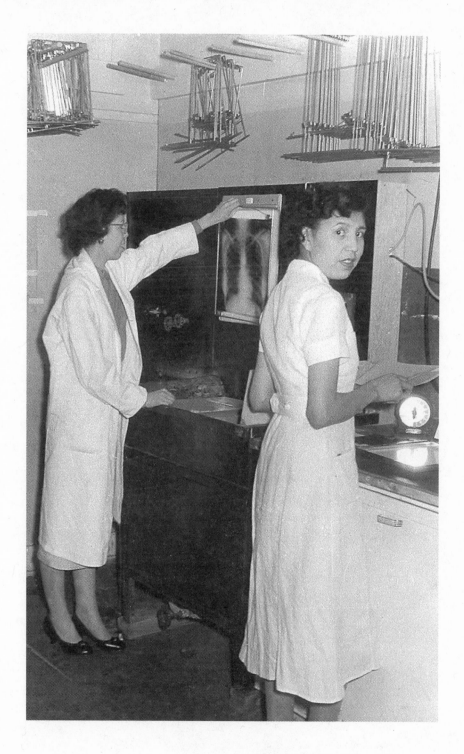

its inception, no records of this program remain beyond documented oral histories of the instructors.[28]

From the IHS perspective, the government was being proactive: "Every effort is made to hire Indians and Eskimos. About 15% of the staff are from these ethnic groups. There are as yet no Indian or Eskimo physicians, but there are a few fully trained and registered public health nurses and many more native ward aides. The male native staff serves mainly as technicians, maintenance men, drivers, etc. although in 1961 the first Indian Sanitarian qualified."[29]

At the same time, IHS had a pervasive and deeply rooted notion that viewed Aboriginal peoples as somehow "behind" in their ability to acquire training and employment at higher levels, which did much to undermine any formal nurse training programs under the auspices of the federal government. As late as 1960 the IHS directorate still had this to say about northwestern Aboriginal communities: "The majority of the present adult Indian population is still employable only in the more humble occupations and consequently can only enjoy a low economic level of existence in our modern western society."[30]

Between 1959 and 1961, IHS annual reports make several mentions of the value of introducing Aboriginal school students, recovering hospital patients, and others falling under federal guidance to health care work. In 1959 the directorate reported with pride that it "continued to participate in programs where medical, nursing and physiotherapy students came for a period of experience and Indian girls were screened to assess their suitability as student practical nurses." That same year, eight "Indian girls" from the Qu'Appelle Diocesan School for Girls were entertained at a dinner and shown films related to a discussion of "opportunities in nursing and related fields."[31]

Training and recruiting Aboriginal workers through IHS facilities was apparently the main tactic used by the Department of National Health and Welfare to create an Aboriginal workforce in health care fields. These efforts were sporadic and unsystematic. This lack of a cohesive approach might be attributed, in part, to the federal government's resistance to creating a "separate" Aboriginal health care system. The principle consistently expressed by the Department of National Health and Welfare through IHS was that "[i]t is not desirable to maintain hospitals purely for Indians if this can be avoided as this tends to perpetuate ideas about Indians being a peculiar people distinct from other Canadians."[32]

Training Aboriginal Nurses and Caregivers

After the Second World War, the federal government launched a number of initiatives to train or encourage Aboriginal peoples to assume para-professional or professional positions within IHS facilities. As early as 1939, small and inconsistent efforts were made to train Native peoples in "nursing" positions via federally supported hospitals, and later as nurses' aides, orderlies, and other technical positions. Mission hospitals supported by Indian Affairs initiated some training efforts, while later IHS hospitals and provincial institutes offered additional opportunities. By the 1960s, IHS involved local community members by training them as community health aides, sanitation aides, and Native health workers.

The IHS system was not the only one offering training in nursing to Aboriginal people. Throughout the twentieth century—and especially after the Second World War—enterprising Native women sought out professionally accredited nurse training in various public facilities. Although financing advanced education was a challenge for these women, some were able to achieve registered nurse designation through their own efforts.

At this time some Canadian schools refused to allow visible minorities to enrol in their nursing programs, therefore, it was not unusual for Aboriginal women to enter nurse training programs in the United States, which were more open to women of colour. As a result, some First Nations women left Canada and moved to the United States to pursue an education in health care.

For example, Wilma Major, of Ojibway-European descent, left hospital training in Ontario for a program in Chicago, where she "was just another minority."[33] Charlotte Monture, of the Six Nations Reserve in southern Ontario, graduated with honours as a registered nurse in 1914 from New Rochelle Hospital School of Nursing in New Rochelle, New York. Mrs. Monture financed her nurse training by taking on a variety of jobs. Following graduation, she continued to work in the state of New York as a public health nurse. She returned to her home reserve in 1921 to marry, raise a family, and continue nursing part-time at the local Indian hospital—the Lady Willingdon Hospital.[34]

Other First Nations women graduated from Canadian institutions before the end of the Second World War. For example, Elizabeth Hill graduated from the Ottawa Civic Hospital in 1933 and subsequently worked at both the Fort Qu'appelle Indian Hospital (Saskatchewan), and the Lady Willingdon Hospital on the Six Nations Reserve. Ruth Porter graduated from Victoria Hospital in London, Ontario, in 1941 and, after working there for some time, moved to the Lady Willingdon Hospital.

Irene Desjarlais of Saskatchewan travelled to Brandon, Manitoba, to receive her RN diploma from the Brandon General Hospital in 1945. Mrs. Desjarlais's career was long and included serving as head nurse at the Fort Qu'appelle Indian Hospital starting in 1953 and eventually becoming the nurse-in-charge and then assistant zone nursing officer within the Medical Services branch in the 1970s.[35] After the war, others followed in the footsteps of these women and entered nurse training at various provincial institutions.

One of Canada's most prominent First Nations nurses was Jean Cuthand Goodwill. Like the other women, she sought her nursing accreditation through a public program at Holy Family Hospital in Prince Albert, Saskatchewan. Graduating in 1954, she became the first Aboriginal person to finish a nursing program in Saskatchewan. She, too, began her career at the Indian hospital at Fort Qu'appelle and later accepted the position of head nurse at IHS's La Ronge nursing station in northern Saskatchewan. Ms. Cuthand Goodwill served in many important leadership roles, including as a member of the board of directors of the Canadian Public Health Association, as

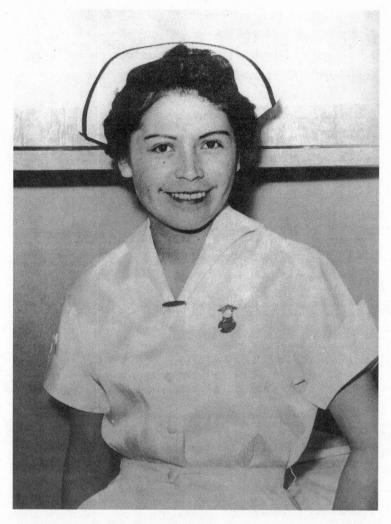

Jean Cuthand Goodwill, Aboriginal nurse. Ms. Cuthand Goodwill became the
first Aboriginal person to finish a nursing program in Saskatchewan. She
later co-founded the Indian and Inuit Nurses of Canada (now known as the
Aboriginal Nurses Association of Canada). [PAA PR1969.0073/MI]

nursing consultant for the Medical Services division, and as special
advisor to the minister of National Health and Welfare.[36]

Many First Nations registered nurses, although trained in public
schools of nursing, eventually took up employment in Indian Health

Services facilities, either in the Indian hospitals or in field nursing work. Some of these nurses were drawn to IHS positions because of the connection to Aboriginal communities and patients. Still, some Aboriginal RNs took positions in provincial service, thereby becoming invisible in the archival record.

Despite the very few IHS-sponsored training opportunities in nursing-related work, Aboriginal registered nurses were hired and working in the Charles Camsell Hospital from an early date. These women were not trained through IHS; rather, they independently pursued their education at established nurse training programs in non-IHS hospitals.

Kathleen Steinhauer of Saddle Lake First Nation was one such nurse. As a young woman she was a guest at the Camsell for the many social functions held for patients, family, and visitors at the hospital. She remembered: "There was no Native Friendship Centre in those days, of course, so for us, the Camsell became the nearest thing to it."

Initially Steinhauer worked for several weeks as a ward aide at the hospital. On her own initiative, she then went on to complete RN training at the nearby Lamont Hospital, graduating in 1954. From there, she worked as an RN at the Camsell, only to be taken aback by some of the circumstances she encountered:

> After I graduated with my RN designation, I went to work in the Indian hospital in Edmonton. That was the Camsell, and I started on the pediatric ward. The conditions there were pretty bad. The babies were all dried with the same towel! I had to petition hard to get separate towels and towel racks for each baby patient. Some things were just improper.[37]

She also recalled being confronted with racism among the nursing staff, though she developed friendships with many of the mostly immigrant maintenance staff employed in the facility.[38] According to other former Aboriginal employees of IHS hospitals, this was not unusual—they all encountered a distinct staff hierarchy and a clear divide between Aboriginal and non-Aboriginal staff. As Kathleen Steinhauer observed, "There was a lot of racism, the staff could be quite patronizing....[T]hey didn't recognize our worth."[39] Violet Clark of Ahousat First Nation, who worked in records at the Nanaimo Indian Hospital, recalled, "The two groups just didn't mingle....[T]hat's just the way it was...maybe we just ignored each other."[40]

In her discussion of nurse training in Canada between the 1940s and 1960s, historian Kathryn McPherson reveals how older patterns of nurse training and work kept it the domain of Caucasian Euro-American women, despite the fact that the need for graduate nurses expanded dramatically during and after the wars. As Jean Cuthand Goodwill, herself an Aboriginal nurse, noted in 1989, First Nations nurses "have faced discrimination and lack of support in the Canadian educational and health care system" and many lacked the financial ability to pursue higher education.[41] Over the years, racial and ethnic barriers facing visible minority women attempting to enter the nursing profession began eroding, even if only gradually.

Although the Canadian Nurses' Association in 1944 reaffirmed its commitment to "support the principle that there be no discrimination in the selection of students for enrolment into schools of nursing," the reality was that some nurse training programs and provincial associations were less than keen on accepting "non-white" members into their midst.[42] Minority women who did enter Canadian nurse training programs, according to Kathryn McPherson, found that their small numbers and ongoing prejudice made the experience a painful one.[43]

Contrary to other Aboriginal health care workers' experiences with racism and underappreciation, Ellen White, a beloved Elder, author, and teacher of the Snuneymuxw First Nation, who was trained in traditional medicine, was recognized for her skills by a doctor at the Nanaimo Indian Hospital. The physician obviously appreciated First Nations peoples as capable health care workers. She recalled, "Dr. Schmidt used me a lot. He was always encouraging me, and came down to the reserve. He encouraged some of us from the reserve to train as health aides."[44]

Training Community Health Workers

Informally, discussion about First Nations community health services began in the late 1950s. At the 1957 annual IHS conference, Ms. Carolyn Dauk, the IHS supervisor of nursing services for Saskatchewan, organized an "environmental sanitation" panel discussion.[45] For the first time, IHS and Indian Affairs representatives involved in health care openly discussed ways to improve the sanitation situation on reserves, including cleaning up water supplies and improving housing. At the end of the conference, the government officials concluded that education was the only way to address the "slum" conditions that existed on reserves.[46] To help with this much-needed education, an "adult education officer" was appointed by Indian Affairs to deal with the situation, and IHS field nurses were directed to approach the government if they needed help improving conditions. The idea of training local Aboriginal community members to improve their own conditions had still to be considered.

Beginning in the 1960s, IHS began to shift its "community health" focus to the training of Aboriginal health care workers, and less on training "nurses" or aides in hospitals. At first, it kept health care delivery and education in the hands of its almost exclusively non-Native staff—especially IHS field nurses. Subsequently, Indian policy began to emphasize "community development" and the Department of National Health and Welfare's IHS launched programs to train Aboriginal peoples to take on public health service responsibilities within their own communities, rather than within IHS facilities. Such programs included the creation of health and welfare committees in Native communities and training "Native health workers"— individuals located in a community who could become assistants and helpers to IHS public health nurses as either sanitation aides or community health aides. A later development was the Indian Health Liaison Officer Program (1969). For IHS, this shift in focus was paramount. As the directorate noted, "Great stress is now being laid on involving the people themselves in discussing and planning solutions of their problems."[47]

Involving Aboriginal peoples in community health work gained
a stronghold. Perhaps the most visible of the community-based
health-training initiatives was the Native Health Worker program. A
sanitation aide training pilot project was run under this new program
in 1960. It involved training twenty-nine delegates—men and women
alike—from the Ohsweken Reserve, near Brantford, Ontario. Chosen
by their band councils, these individuals received training in issues
related to sanitation at IHS's Lady Willingdon Hospital. Assisted by
a regional sanitarian and health educator, the workshop aimed to
educate toward improving sanitation on reserves. The workshop
was well received by the participants, and IHS concluded, "we have
learned that the workshop technique, an unknown quantity in this
particular setting, is a workable and effective method of stimulating
interest in and action on local problems."[48]

Next, the Community Health Auxiliary (CHA) course, launched in
1961, became the more prominent of the two Native Health Worker
programs. In that year, the first course for CHA was held in Norway
House in northern Manitoba, co-sponsored by the Department of
Indian Affairs and the Medical Services branch.[49] As with the sanitation aides, local band councils chose who would attend. The first
class consisted of four women and seven men. The program was held
both in the trainees' own communities and at the Norway House
Indian Hospital, and lasted several months. As a group, the students
were introduced to basic health knowledge, germ theory, nutrition,
and first aid. They also went into the field to observe conditions in
Native communities and gain experience in holding public meetings.
Following this general education, the men and women were split up;
the women were subsequently trained in public health nursing techniques, and the men in practical sanitation.[50] From that date forward,
community health worker training programs continued.

Staff did not often articulate the fact that the IHS system
imposed "outside" health care structures and non-Aboriginal staff
on First Nations communities. A few government employees recognized, however, that the creation of community health worker
training programs could serve as the answer to the ills of the IHS

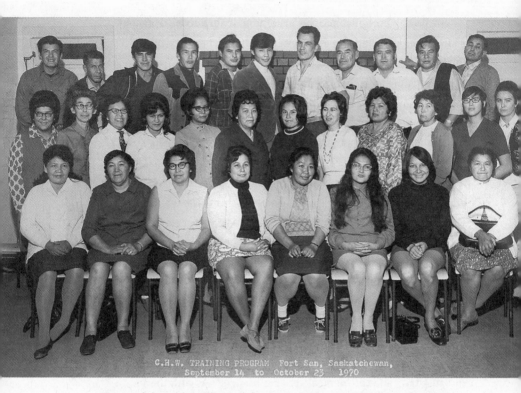

C.H.W. TRAINING PROGRAM Fort San, Saskatchewan,
September 14 to October 23 1970

Community Health Worker Training Program, Fort Qu'Appelle Sanatorium, Saskatchewan, 1970. Indian Health Services offered various opportunities for Aboriginal people to become trained as health care workers. [PAA 91.383.500]

system because, through these programs, Aboriginal health workers could control delivery of community health care. In 1966 Ethel G. Martins, writing for the *Canadian Journal of Public Health* about training Aboriginal health care workers noted, "For years, doctors, nurses and others have been attempting to inculcate public health concepts into Indians and Eskimos with disappointingly meager results....Telling has not worked."[51] "Planned change does not stem from a standard pattern [of health care] proposed at the national level....[P]eople for whom the program is intended must be involved in the planning and implementation."[52]

Surprisingly, as a result of these realizations, IHS launched community health worker training with the aim of bridging "the culture gap" between Medical Services' personnel and their Aboriginal clients.[53] In 1966 Dr. Percy E. Moore enthused,

> A campaign to train native health workers has proved valuable and interesting. Various communities are asked to select a candidate, and a group, so selected are brought to central points, usually where a hospital is located, for example Cambridge Bay. These persons are paid so that the family at home does not suffer if the recruit happens to be the breadwinner. A course of intensive instruction for about three months is given after which the trainees go back to their communities, and are put on salary to work under the direction of the departmental medical or nursing personnel. This program seems to be a successful one.[54]

As ambitious and well-intentioned as the CHA course was, historian Mary Jane McCallum writes, "The training and hiring of CHRS was not an early example of 'affirmative action' in the civil service, as the under-representation of Aboriginal People in the Department of Health and Welfare was only tangentially discussed. This was a dead-end and precarious position relatively low on the Indian Health Services hierarchy, and...was ultimately created with the intention of being phased out to provincial services."[55]

Despite what seems to have been token efforts to include Aboriginal peoples in the IHS system at the community level, prejudice remained among IHS staff. Non-Aboriginal nursing staff continued to believe in their expertise in health matters, and some only grudgingly conceded the "expertise" of Aboriginal community health trainees on matters related to their own communities. As an IHS advisor reflected after participating in community health worker training, "There seems to be a need for more understanding on the part of the nurses of the culture of the natives....[A]lso they should be aware of their own set of beliefs and attitudes."[56]

In contrast, Aboriginal peoples responded enthusiastically to their involvement in community health worker training and did not consider the program as mere tokenism. "Why weren't we told this long ago?" they asked.[57] The seeds for self-determination in Aboriginal health care had been sown.

In a policy memo dated December 2, 1969, the director of Medical Services forecast that federal policy was heading toward increasing

IHS presence in the northern regions of the country, while simultaneously decreasing the federal presence in the southern provinces.
At the same time, liaison arrangements with Aboriginal political
organizations and "progressive" bands would lead to these groups
"taking over some of the administration of health services in their
own areas."[58]

The goal of Medical Services was to reduce its direct involvement
in Aboriginal health care delivery. In the area of training, Medical
Services only directly supported training for Native workers, community health workers, and community aides in both the South
and North. The long-held vision of Indian Health Services—that it
was a service for Aboriginal peoples rather than a service of which
Aboriginal people were a part—lasted well into the 1970s.

The 1970s marked a period of intense debate in Canada over the
nature of federal commitment and involvement with registered Indian
peoples, and all Aboriginal groups generally. The issue of health care
and its formal delivery to Aboriginal communities was very much part
of many of the conversations held by Aboriginal leaders and government representatives at this time. It was always clear, however, that
the federal government would only indirectly encourage the involvement of Aboriginal peoples in its Medical Services at the community
level. The philosophy continued to prevail in Ottawa that Indian,
Métis, and Inuit peoples should receive formal health care in the
same manner as all "other" Canadians, and, at most, would control
the administration themselves. By 1974 Native employees in the
service were at an all-time high—18 per cent of all staff—including
general labour.[59]

Government records suggest that Aboriginal peoples came to
work at IHS through a variety of avenues: as patients in the system
who were subsequently trained to assume IHS technical positions;
as young people selected through the Indian Residential Schools
system; or as individuals hired on at various IHS facilities. Although
it is difficult to generalize, a pattern emerged to reveal indigenous
labour concentrated in the lower levels of the health care worker
hierarchy. Those who did enter into higher levels in IHS only did so by

struggling for a higher education that enabled them to gain professional designations.

Through oral stories, we can better understand the experience of Aboriginal people working within IHS. Aboriginal people describe varied reasons for working at IHS. Some chose health care careers for the stability of a government wage job; some out of personal interest; some were inspired by health care workers whom they encountered as patients in hospital; and still others assumed posts at IHS in order to be closer to their own families who were hospitalized.

As IHS cooks, technicians, orderlies, sanitarians, nurses' aides, practical nurses, community health workers, and registered nurses, Aboriginal peoples represented an important interface between IHS and the Aboriginal communities they served. These workers were the translators, the caretakers, the comforters, and the helpers of Aboriginal patients in a system over which their own communities had little control.

ABORIGINAL NURSE AT THE CAMSELL

Kathleen Steinhauer

Kathleen Steinhauer and her husband, Gilbert Anderson, were the first people I interviewed regarding their experiences with Indian Health Services and, more specifically, Edmonton's Charles Camsell Indian Hospital.

Our initial conversation occurred in 2004. I won't forget how nervous I was arranging the interview and how, when I tried to tape our conversation at their dining room table, I fumbled with dead batteries in my recorder. Taping wouldn't work; listening would. Luckily, Kathleen and Gilbert were very kind and patient.

During short breaks, Gilbert shored up my nerves by playing samples of Métis fiddle music on the stereo and talking about his collection of fiddles, which were lovingly nestled on the couch. He reminded me that music was an important part of life for the patients and their families at Camsell. Patients loved their guitars and radios, and many joined in on the dances that were held now and then. Long conversations with them brought forward the nuances of a hospital

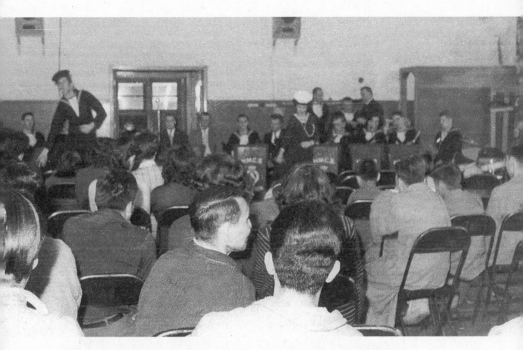

Patients at the Charles Camsell Indian Hospital enjoy visiting entertainers, 1950s. Dances, music, movies and other forms of entertainment were provided for patients in the hospital as their convalescence was typically long and marked by hours of rest and boredom. [PAA 91.383.87]

and health care system that affected so many people in Edmonton and regions North.

Kathleen Steinhauer's stories are very carefully considered and nuanced. Her portrayal of the facility and life within it is never dramatic. She explains the atmosphere of the institution and her work there almost dispassionately. What is absent from her stories, however, is any true enthusiasm for the Camsell. Steinhauer's memories are different from those of Elva Taylor, director of nursing at the Camsell (see page 33 for Elva Taylor's stories about the Camsell).

Ms. Taylor was a mentor for Steinhauer, but the tone of her stories about the nature and quality of care in the hospital are very different. Taylor's memories are about helping, and offer less, if little, insight about the social and emotional dislocation that patients may have felt at the hospital. Taylor speaks from the position of authority. Steinhauer's accounts work like a bridge of understanding, moving back and forth between describing how patients and caregivers struggled with the task confronting them: healing very sick people from many and diverse communities. She could do this because she herself understood the social and cultural backgrounds of those who were in the hospital—workers and patients alike.

~~~~~~~~

I WAS BORN ON THE SADDLE LAKE RESERVE in northeastern Alberta. My father, Ralph Steinhauer, was a farmer there, and when we were young my sisters, brother, and I also worked on the farm. We attended residential school at first, but my parents decided to pull us from that school when I was eight years old. We were home schooled for a short time, and after that we went to the United Church school in Bonnyville. The teachers were nicer there. Once I was finished my elementary schooling, I went to Alberta College in Edmonton in 1947. It was a high school with boarding students from all over. I stayed in the dorms. My grandmother—my mother's mother—lived in Edmonton, so we felt at home there. We couldn't attend our local high school because, as registered Indians, we were not accepted into public school at that time.

One of the things we did in high school was visit the Charles Camsell Hospital. There were lots of familiar people there, and social events like dances and movie nights, and members from the community were welcome to drop in. Sunday visits to the hospital were a popular thing to do. It was our "friendship centre." After high school, I was recruited to work as a ward aide by the director of nursing at the Camsell, Miss Taylor. I did that job for about six weeks.

I was inspired to be a nurse by my Aunt Margaret, my father's brother's wife. My family was always cautious regarding health. We grew up far from any hospital and we didn't have a car. Lots of people died on the reserve when I was young, and I thought, "I want

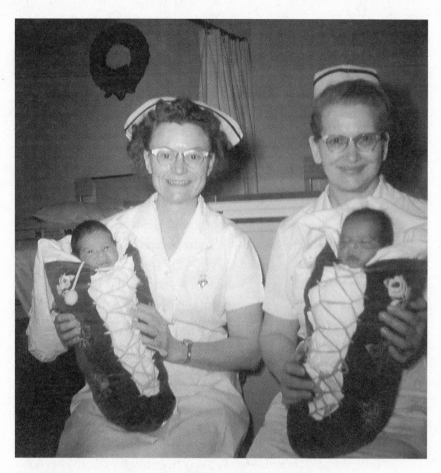

Nurses hold young patients in Charles Camsell Indian Hospital, Edmonton, 1950s. Nurses from the Indian Hospital system recall with fondness their contact with their youngest patients. Not all children survived their illness, and many children and adults were buried in the St. Albert Cemetery, northwest of Edmonton, or at the Edmonton Indian Residential School cemetery. [PAA 91.383.154]

to be a doctor, then I would help." There was so little help for Indian people in those days. Of course, people on reserve continued to use traditional health and healing techniques, but they mostly did this secretly and privately.

At first I thought I was going to be a doctor, but when I saw the doctors I knew I didn't think I had that kind of confidence at the time. At Saddle Lake, where my Aunt Margaret worked as nurse, there was no nursing station. She lived at the Indian agent's house and she had an old car. I was seventeen when I first met her, and she was engaged to my uncle. She had a scrapbook she used to show us about her nursing training. Her father wanted her to go into insurance, but she only lasted for a year. In the middle of her training she contracted tuberculosis, and she had to take time off before going back to nursing. My aunt was a public health nurse, and later she encouraged me to be a public health nurse, too, since she thought it was a good schedule for someone with children.

I started my nurse training in the small town of Lamont, outside Edmonton. There was a United Church hospital there, and I began training for my RN as part of a class of thirteen students. We graduated in 1954. We wrote our exams in September, and the girls from university hospitals who were writing the exams at the same time didn't pay much attention to us country girls. We thought they were quite snobbish, but that didn't bother us—we were convinced we had a good chance to pass. Those others didn't pass, and we had a hard time biting our tongues!

As soon as I finished school, my first job was working at the Camsell. I started in the children's ward and dealt mostly with babies for about eighteen months. I remember that hospital was not a rich facility when I started there. You have to remember that the Camsell was a tuberculosis hospital to begin with.

When I first started working with the babies, I noticed they were drying them all with the same towels. It was shocking to me, and so I petitioned to have each child have their own towel on their own separate rack.

Indian hospitals were not really a popular place to work, although the pay was pretty good. There was a shortage of staff in these hospitals, especially nurses, and those that were there were often old or unsuitable. After that first eighteen months I requested a transfer to another Indian hospital—the Blood Indian Hospital at Cardston in southern Alberta. I knew some girls from that reserve who were my age and working. Unfortunately, I became quite sick down there, and they sent me back to Edmonton. Eventually I returned, and I worked in Cardston for three years. From Cardston I moved around to the Indian hospital at Hobbema, then Pincher Creek, and finally I decided to try to return home.

I applied to work as a nurse at Saddle Lake, but because that was my home community, they turned me down. My Aunt Marg came to the rescue, and she hired me at the St. Paul health unit in the summer of 1960. That was the start of my switch to public health nursing.

In 1960 I started my training in public health nursing. I obtained a provincial government bursary that year to attend the University of Alberta and train for one academic year. I completed my field training in Cranbrook, British Columbia. I really enjoyed public health—I didn't feel confined, and I finally felt like I was *preventing* illness. From there I worked in the provincial health service for four years, and then I moved to work for the City of Edmonton, in public health again.

Although I started my nursing career in the Charles Camsell Indian Hospital, it wasn't until 1972 that I came back to it. My old friend Joe Atkinson, an R N for the Indian Health Service, saw me at the Camsell one day and he enticed me to take a position in "patient transportation" at the Camsell. In this role, I was responsible for arranging patient transportation from the hospital, making sure patients got back home if they lived out of town, and sometimes I served as a patient escort. It was an interesting job, and although it was a clerk position, I found it challenging.

When I worked in the Camsell as a registered nurse, Aboriginal people worked in various jobs within the institution. But there were not many other Aboriginal R Ns. I remember Jennie Tallow was an R N. There were several Aboriginal nursing aides, however. People like Sylvia Fox and Rosie Tailfeathers. Girls that wanted to become nursing aides could take their training in Calgary or Edmonton. This training fell under provincial control, and took ten months to complete.

Besides nursing aides, Aboriginal people worked in the laundry, as cooking and cleaning staff. Some were also orderlies or reception-ists. I recall that patients in the hospital sometimes became staff and workers, as well, once they'd recovered. Not everyone thought of their work in the hospital as especially good or unique. For many people, working in the hospital was just a job. As an RN, I worked long hours. Luckily our matron, Mrs. Rapley, and our director of nursing, Miss Taylor, were very dedicated. Miss Taylor started a maternity ward in the Camsell, for example, since although the hospital was for tuberculosis treatment, there were pregnant women who arrived there, and some women even became pregnant in hospital.

For Aboriginal people recovering from tuberculosis, their stay in the Camsell was a real trial. I think that some of the staff understood. But there were a lot of staff who were tough, and were not particularly sympathetic. There were patients who couldn't speak English, and there were not many well people who could translate. They had no trouble with Cree speakers since there were enough Cree speakers around in the hospital to translate. Still, language barriers were a daily challenge.

The treatment and the hospital were also very confining for people. I recall a fellow from Saddle Lake—he would escape from the Camsell and the police would bring him back. The police had the power to bring him back. Under the Indian Act, someone who has tuberculosis could be apprehended for treatment. Once, word spread around the hospital that the police had recaptured the gentlemen from Saddle Lake and that he was back at the Camsell. There was a little cubicle on the roof of the hospital building and they said it was the jail. I never saw it but I did hear about it. He was kept there, in bed and under guard.

There were many displaced persons—DPs—from the Second World War who worked at the hospital, and one of these DPs was appointed to look after the jailbird. One night we heard a terrible crash. The first thing the nurse on the children's ward thought was that one of the children had fallen out of their bed. She put on the lights in the ward and looked out of the window. What did she see? She saw that man, in his pyjamas, jumping on the tin roof, running out of there.

In some ways, the Camsell was like a jail. The patients couldn't leave. Today, hospitals are very different and tuberculosis is treated very differently. There are medications that people can take at home. Back then, bed rest was strictly enforced, and the treatments were sometimes surgical. During their convalescence, many patients were too weak to get out of bed, and some never recovered their strength. Some were in the hospital for years.

Many patients arrived at the Camsell as infants and grew up in the institution. Of course, family members could visit their relatives, and there were places visitors could stay at the Camsell, but for many the hospital was too far away to visit with any frequency. Tragically, not all the bodies of those who succumbed to their illness were returned home. Bodies were returned home by train, if possible, otherwise they were buried at the Enoch Reserve. The St. Albert cemetery has a monument to these individuals.

There is a thought that the hospitals were used for medical experiments. Occasionally new treatments for tuberculosis emerged and it seemed to many people, including patients and staff, that these treatments were pioneered on patients in the Indian Hospital system. When patients consented to treatment, I believe they often did not fully understand what was being asked of them.

When I first started working at the Camsell as an RN, I recall feeling uncomfortable at times. Nurses in the residence sometimes made inappropriate comments about the Indian patients, and that was upsetting to me. Many of the non-Native staff wanted to be in control all the time, only do things their way. I thought these people could be quite patronizing, never acknowledging the worth of their Aboriginal staff or colleagues. In fact, racism was common inside the hospital.

Even today, many of the former staff do not understand the point of view of Aboriginal people. After all these years, I believe very strongly that the patients shouldn't have had to go to the Charles Camsell Hospital.

NANAIMO INDIAN HOSPITAL—
BEING A PATIENT AND BECOMING A NURSE
Michael Dick

Michael Dick and his wife, Marie, both spent time sharing stories about their experiences in the Indian Hospital system. I visited them at their home in Nanaimo, and they spoke at length while we drank coffee and family members dropped by to visit and listen. Michael is an expert storyteller, and it was very important to him to tell his story by linking it to his childhood, for his time in hospital was his childhood. Today he is a proud advocate of First Nations education, and someone who is eager to have the details of his experience shared. "Tell everyone!" were his words to me.

Michael's account emphasizes how important it was to him to survive and make something of himself. He knew his opportunities were limited, yet he was determined to be successful and make a living. The Indian hospital provided him with opportunities, but also coloured his life experience and opened his eyes to what he felt were blatant inequities in society. Despite that, he is proud of his long and dedicated career as a caregiver.

THIS IS MY STORY. IT STARTS IN THE YEAR there was a flood in my home community of Kingcome Inlet, on the north coast of British Columbia. It was one of those floods where the watermark went right into the houses, and the people were taken out. Not everyone left. Certain individuals who were still in their homes stayed but moved to higher ground. They knew my mother was pregnant and ready to deliver so they went to get her in this canoe. The canoe went right into the house, alongside her bed, and she was moved over into the canoe, moving out to higher ground. That was where I was born!

I did not have a name at that time. I did not have a name for a long time. I eventually became named Michael. I eventually also got my Indian name in the presence of the big house. Growing up, I remember singing our traditional songs under the kitchen table. But it didn't seem a long time before I was taken by some people to go to school.

The next thing I recall is arriving at this island, where the residential school was. It was St. Michael's Indian Residential School at Alert Bay. At this time my dad was a fisherman, so I would go down to the corner of the fence, on the grounds, looking out, waiting for my dad because I didn't know what I was there for. So I stayed there probably four years.

During my tenure at that boarding school for three or four years—I don't know because at that age you can't be very precise—I remember being picked up, picked up off the floor. I remember that I was fainting. I was taken to a preventorium, which was on the premises of the residential school. There we were bedridden—we weren't allowed out of bed. I dropped my pencil, I remember, and I got up to retrieve it. That is one thing that I remember so vividly—the nurse tore the living hell out of me for getting out of bed. You see, at that age I thought, "Why am I in bed?" I didn't know. I remember I said something back to that nurse, for which he gave me one good licking! If I recall correctly, I said to him, "My brother is in the war— what are you doing here?" I remember that. The words that come out of babes' mouths!

So, I can't recall the length of time I spent there, whether it was a year or two years, but it was long. Then one day I left. I was escorted out of that building by a Caucasian man—he took me on a ship. It was an overnight trip, I remember that, and when we got to our destination, I was surprised by the lights. I had never seen so many lights, I didn't know where I was, or what all these lights were! When we arrived he took me in a car, and we went up the hill, to buildings which were barracks. This was the Indian hospital.

I was all by myself. I was probably around seven or eight years old, something like that. We went up to the barracks. And in that building were all of these men. They were soldiers shipping out for Halifax. My brother was there. So I stayed there. There were maybe four buildings. Outside was a light that was on all night long. We were not supposed to be outside at night. Or out of bed.

In the hospital, the individuals that worked there had different ways of gaining our respect. Their demeanour was individual. That's not to say there weren't nice people. There were. I stayed in the cubicle, in my bed, and I would cover myself up with my blanket and sing to myself in my own language, over and over again. I would also talk to my mom and family and answer for them at night. That's how I kept my language. The kid across from me in another bed, he died.

I stayed there perhaps five years. When I was around thirteen I was schooled. I don't know if the teachers were volunteers, but there was a lady called Mary Brown, and a nurse named Mrs. King. They seemed to like me.

I saw a lot of stuff. I saw a lot of what they, the staff, did. Eventually after seeing all these things, the revelation to my mind was more pronounced there at that time. I was now asking myself questions. I was now seeing how patients were treated, and that things were not right. I didn't question it when I was younger, but I did now. I had swollen glands. I took PAS, INH, streptomycin.

I saw people coming out of a certain room, where they had had their lungs collapsed. That was called a pneumothorax. As I understand it, they insert a tube into the chest to collapse the lung. The belief was that a pneumothorax would rest the lung. I didn't know all this at the time, but later I learned about it by learning anatomy and physiology. They also used to do gastric lavages. I suppose that was the only way they could culture the sputum. They were painful procedures, not pleasant at all. And there wasn't any sedation or painkillers, other than aspirins. Reflecting on it now, I truly believe to some degree there was a lot of medical pioneering going on.

After a few years, it was time for me to go home. Upon my arrival back home, I could see that things were different there now. My relationship with my family, the closeness I had had as a child, was missing. I had been away for so long. I missed that bonding. The close relationship with my family was taken away by my time in the school and the hospital. I could see that despite the fact that things weren't right, I could see it. Maybe I saw it more than others.

So there I was, home. And now I was now a teenager. I went home for four years. I took off into the wilderness. I wanted to get away from people, and I spent a lot of time by myself. I knew there was something wrong. This was my journey. They did TB surveys at that time, and when I got checked it turned out I wasn't better. I had to go back to the hospital.

When I returned, Mary Brown was still there. It was just like starting over in there. I don't know whatever drugs they used, but I think they were the same drugs. There I stayed for probably three or four more years. During my convalescence, they got me on steroids and exercise. They had a 16mm projector, for films, and I would go from ward to ward showing movies. They were just common movies. Cowboys shootin' up Indians! I don't recall seeing any health movies. I'd never ran a projector before, but I ran that machine up there! So I was still going to school. I couldn't go back home.

They also allowed me to work, first wiping tables, and later running the sterilizing equipment. I even saw an appendectomy. I was masked, gowned, and I stood on a stool to watch the first appendectomy at NIH [Nanaimo Indian Hospital]. I was gaining some basic skills. I also saw patients get upset. I remember vividly how for one fellow it was too much. You have to understand that there was no social worker at that facility to make things smoother for the patients.

Then one day I discovered I had two sisters. And I didn't know for how long! She was one of the two girls who, when I was at that preventorium at residential school when I was so young, I saw waving at me. At that time, so many years ago I didn't know who they were. They were both my sisters! They were younger than me. There are two sisters and three brothers in my family.

I won't go into detail about all that I saw, all the things that sometimes went on. But these people I remember watching, they were all grown-up people. I felt so sorry for one guy. He just had a breakdown. He was thrashing around. He was begging to end it all. I can remember a few guys like that. They would send orderlies in to deal with patients like that. The staff knew that I spoke my language, and so they asked me to help with this one individual. So I went and I spoke to him.

I knew, deep inside of me, what was wrong. But the whole process, the interaction was wrong. It wasn't about caring; the whole interaction between patients and staff wasn't about caring. It wasn't about that. The doctors and nurses were all hardcore Europeans. We heard so many racist comments. One of the orderlies, his last name was Krauss. He was in the Hitler ranks, and he made no bones about it! These were hardened people. There were lots of negative things. There were more negative aspects than there were positive to our time in the hospital.

Then I went home for the second time. At that time, Mary Brown asked me to fill out a form. She actually insisted. Because she was so nice to me, I did it. She was the nicest person I knew up there in the hospital. I knew I could trust her. She and another nurse were probably the only ones I really trusted. I went back to Kingcome Inlet for about six months. It seems like a short time, but then I received a letter to come and work at the hospital, as an orderly. That was in 1953. I worked at NIH for ten years.

There were written exams at NIH, which was the protocol for my being in the capacity that I was. When I was an orderly I was told what my parameters were, and that's how I worked there.

Then, in 1963, I received a phone call from the director of nursing at the Nanaimo Regional General Hospital (NRGH). They had just opened and I was asked to work there. I was very lucky. What I didn't know was that Mary Brown was working on my behalf. She knew the director of nursing. I finally accepted. Later I found out that every year she checked on how I was doing, without my knowing. I was hired as an orderly, but my job was not limited. I was learning all kinds of things. I learned that the nursing care in the regular hospital was very different than in the Indian hospital. Even though they had a program and people wrote exams to work at NIH, when I got to NRGH I saw the difference in the standards. Standards at the NIH were lower.

When I work in NRGH in 1976, they asked me to continue my studies as a practical nurse. Things were going so well for me, I was chosen to go back and help teach skill sets and with career choices for students. I was advancing in my career and continued to be an advocate of it, too! I saw nursing at its best! It was not long after I started working at NRGH, I saw all kinds of people from all parts of the world and all kinds of backgrounds. And I worked with them.

I worked for thirty years as a practical nurse. I have my original practical nurse pin from 1975! The first thirteen years of my nursing career were on the ward. Then I went into emergency, as there was an opening there. My work was not much different from a general duty nurse; in those days it was not specialized. Now it has become quite specialized. It became quite specialized over the years that I was working.

There weren't too many in my generation that went into nursing. I never had a chance to choose. I had to survive, and the only way that I could see that I could survive was to go along with Mary Brown. From the get-go it was like, my mother never mothered me per se, but it was like with Mary Brown, it was sort of like that. It gave me some security. I felt safe.

My mother once came to see Mary Brown. My mom went to this church behind Departure Bay, and there was a lady at the door greeting, and this lady noticed my mom, who had never been in that building. So the lady went to greet my mom. The greeter was Mary Brown! Mary asked my mother if she knew Michael Dick, and my mother looked up at this lady and said, "He's my son."

Mary paused, and said, "He's my son, too." I didn't know about this—it was somebody else that heard their conversation and told me about it.

I think my parents came down maybe twice to see me. I wrote letters to my family, but I knew I wouldn't be getting any answers anyway, because my mom and dad didn't write. My mom and dad were dedicated to the church, as well as to our traditional rituals.

I went to see Dr. Rob Lee when I was sick, and it cost five bucks. And he said, "Why are you seeing me here, when you have your own hospital up the hill?" I told him point blank, "The care up there is really bad."

The staff in our Indian hospital were not all bad, there were some good people, but I know there were racists there. They would have parties and never invite the Indian workers. The nurses were separate from everyone else. There was no mingling. I remember it being a hot topic when the first Indian joined the nurses at a party. I remember it being discussed as a very hot topic. The dialogue that went on! These were the days when we still sat at the back of the bus! [laughs] We used to go to the movie theatre and they would put us upstairs! It is no different. They were supposedly caregivers.

The same type of caregivers were in the residential school. They were supposed to be caregivers for health and education. They didn't do a good job. I got sick at school. When I came here [to the Nanaimo Indian Hospital], it just extended the same thing that I was dealing with at school. It was the same thing. The same tree, and that tree has deep roots. Looking back at the stuff they did, I can't prove it in court, but I am positive that there was experimentation. If you remember the Thalidomide crisis—in my mind that's the same category. I heard rumours of the hospital closing in '64 or '65, and I think it closed in '69 or so. I went to NRGH in 1963.

WARD AIDE AND OFFICE ASSISTANT AT THE NANAIMO INDIAN HOSPITAL

Violet Clark

Violet Clark worked in the Nanaimo Indian Hospital as a young woman. One day, while in conversation with Delores Louie, she discovered that Delores was helping to research the history of the Nanaimo Indian Hospital, and she volunteered to be interviewed. Delores Louie, Violet Clark, and I met at the White Spot restaurant to record Violet's memories of her work at the hospital. At first she thought she couldn't really remember that much. Then, as she spoke, the memories came back to her. At the end of our interview, she laughed and said, "The more I talk to you, the more I remember. Some of these things I hadn't thought about for years!" Sometimes an audience is key to helping a storyteller remember.

Violet Clark portrayed life in the hospital in a matter-of-fact manner. Her even-tempered and non-judgmental recollections of the difficult aspects of hospital life—the frustrations of patients, the painful treatments, and the social and professional divisions between Aboriginal and non-Aboriginal workers within the hospital system—in some ways belie the traumatic impact of these realities on many of those who experienced them. As an employee in the hospital, she was insulated from the immediate pain felt by so many very ill patients. Yet, she reminds us how compliant people were at this time and how most people, it seems, accepted how hard things were for them. Her story leaves room for and invites us to imagine life in these complex institutions, for workers and patients alike.

~~~~~~~~~~~~~

I'M FROM AHOUSAT AND MY NAME IS VIOLET CLARK. I attended the Indian residential school in Port Alberni for thirteen years, and that's how I got working in the Nanaimo Indian Hospital. I worked there for the summers when I was sixteen, seventeen, and eighteen. Then I worked there year-round when I was nineteen and twenty. I got out of residential school in 1953, just before my twentieth birthday.

I worked as a maid in the hospital for the first three years and then—I don't know what happened—I had real bad chest congestion all of the time, so they took me out of the wards and put me in the office. They treated me with sunlamps, although at the time I didn't know what those lamps were for. After that, I had X-rays and they tested me, which showed that I had been in contact with tuberculosis. For twenty-four months I worked in the hospital office, transcribing for doctors.

There were quite a few different offices in the hospital. In the office I was in, there was just me, and I worked only four hours in the afternoon because I was getting treatment in the morning. I lived right at the hospital until the last weeks I was there, when I got an apartment with a friend who worked at the hospital. From there I followed my parents to the States. So, I worked there three summers and then in the office. I left the hospital in 1954.

There is a connection between the residential schools and the hospitals.

The principal of the Alberni Residential School was influential in linking the school and the hospital. He wanted young people to go and work. I wasn't the only student from Alberni Residential School to get hired on at the hospital. The first year, Frieda Maitland, Hannah Little, and a girl named Ruby from Kitimat were hired part-time. In fact, several girls from the school were hired. I knew a few of them from Duncan. It was mostly girls, but one year there was one fellow. He did orderly jobs or whatever. I thought it was a good opportunity.

I know my father was not so keen on my working there. He thought I was too young to go out on my own, since I was only sixteen. The school had made arrangements for the hospital and he wasn't sure we were looked after properly. So Dad sent my brother down to pick me up. I sure felt caught in the middle! The principal of the school told me it was going to be a good experience, but my dad didn't want me to do it. In the end, it was my decision, and I chose against my dad. To make up for my decision, I went home every summer for the last two weeks to visit my family. That made my parents feel better.

Eventually Dad was glad that I did work there. I had an older sister who worked at the hospital for a little while, and then she transferred to the Coqualeetza Indian Hospital. From Coqualeetza, she went to work in Vancouver in a public hospital. I don't know what my father was thinking. Maybe he was worried that I would wander around like my sister. But she was ten years older than me. I am glad I worked at the hospital. I don't know what I would have done if I'd stayed at home on the reserve in Ahousat.

They generally started you as a ward maid. Our uniform looked like a nurse's uniform, but it was blue, light blue, and maybe some green. It was a shift dress, some with buttons all the way down. Our job was to do cleaning. We would also help the kitchen people serve a meal, or help a patient move a bed, or conversations with patients. We got to know them well. We could make friends with the patients. They couldn't stop us!

Every Thursday evening the staff was allowed to go visit family and friends or whomever you wanted in the hospital. There were quite a few patients from Ahousat that I knew. I made a point of trying to visit people I knew. I also tried to walk through the wards because a lot of people didn't get visitors, and just say "hullo" and chat with them. Nearly all the workers did that. They would make a point to do the visiting on Thursdays.

The hospital had a nurses' home. The nurses and aides all lived there, since room and board were provided. There were over twenty or thirty people living there. The nurses and the aides were a mix of Aboriginal and non-Aboriginal people. The Aboriginal people were all aides, not nurses. The Aboriginal aides lived in one wing and the non-Native nurses in the other wing. We had our own bedroom, very small. It was above the hospital. They were barracks, just like the hospital. The doctors' building was right next door. The doctors had the same set-up as we had.

We worked so hard, and it was so hot in the summers here! We used to laugh about it. Some of us would shower three times a day just to cool off, eh. In the breaks, we would do that. We must've put in long hours. More than eight hours in a shift, I think. It was pretty good with the aides that I worked with. I used to feel sorry for the patients in the summer especially. People were roasting in wards. I used to feel really bad for them. It was so hot. There was no air conditioning. Patients were not allowed outside, as far as I knew. Maybe later patients were allowed outside.

All I could think of was "work, work, work." We worked from 6 a.m. until 10 a.m. in the morning, and then go back at 2 p.m. and finish about 6:30 or 7 p.m. in the evening. I have no idea what I made in wages. I got a cheque at the end of each month. But I kept all my cheques until the end of my work period!

There was not a lot of turnover in staff. There was a friendly nurse the last year I was there. She used to invite us to her home on Prideaux Street. Quite often. For a meal or to just come for the evening and play games. There was also one doctor who was really, really good to the young people. Dr. Ewing. He took us, four young people, to dinner in Duncan. We were all aide workers, all from Alberni school. He took us to a very nice restaurant, and we were sitting there with him when the waiter came and said, "I'm sorry, we can't serve you. I need you to sit in the back." This is what the waiter told the doctor. It was strange!

The doctor really apologized to us and wanted to leave. This was in the early 1950s. My goodness! That was my first really strange experience. The waiter was really good—he brought a lady along, and the doctor talked to her—the manager—and so we had to sit at separate tables from the doctor, but we did sit close together. We ate dinner and carried on our conversation! He was a very helpful person, that doctor. Other doctors, well, we just ignored each other. Very few were very friendly. We just ignored the unfriendly ones.

The doctors and the nurses all ate in a different dining room than we did. And there were non-Natives sitting with us, too, but they were all maids and orderlies and like that. The one New Year's that I was there, the doctors made a point to come and sit with all the workers. A few sat at each table and tried to mingle.

On the wards, the mood was often up and down. Some days you'd go to work and patients would be upbeat, and some days the mood was so dismal. Nobody was there for just a few months; people were there for a long time. Many couldn't walk past the doorway. The wards were quite big. I don't know how many patients in each, but there were four patients in each cubicle, four beds. The walls were only halfway to the ceiling, so patients could talk to each other. As a patient, you could walk out of your cubicle, but you would have to stick in the area. People couldn't go outside.

I used to feel really bad, once a month when they would get their needles, whatever it was. Oh, they would line them up in the hallway, way down the other end where we could hardly see the people, and we could hear them moaning and groaning. They would have to sit there until the pain subsided, and only then would someone escort them back to the wards. All that moaning and groaning is what I remember most. It locks in your memory forever. I used to be so curious to see what was going on. Then the patients would tell us how painful the needles were. The smell was always there, too. It was probably because of the medication of the patients, and many patients had sores. No matter how much you cleaned that hospital, it always had a smell.

It was like a community inside the hospital. It's really amazing. I recall males asking us to deliver letters to the ladies! How those men ever got the name of a girl, or knew what they looked like, I don't know, but they had pictures on the walls of their girls. "Bring this to that girl!" they'd say. It sure was strange! Actually, I remember being shocked at one case I remember. This man was a patient in the hospital, and he was married with quite a few children. Yet, in the hospital over here, he was right into another girl. Eventually he married that girl from the hospital.

Now that I think about it, I don't think there was a way for patients to get hold of their own clothing. There were no storage areas. I remember they just had these little nightstands. I don't know where they put their clothes. The hospital gave them pyjamas or nightgowns. But then some of the ladies had their own housecoats and bed jackets. So I guess they were allowed some of their own bedclothes.

It was a very regimented day in the hospital. They had a poor library—the women on their side. Just had a few little rows of books and magazines. They were allowed to go to the library to get a book. Patients got a pass to get a book. I never saw any teachers, but I heard that they did do that. Not so much high school, but for the elementary kids. My cousin, Doris, she was at the residential school for only a week when they sent her to the hospital. So she went to school for seven years while she was in the hospital.

When I got sick and was moved to office work, I got blood tests and X-rays, and they gave me times for treatments. I'd go and do what they told me. I would let myself get treated with sunlamps and some kind of lights. They never explained the treatment to me. All I knew was that it had to do with my chest congestion. There was no real explanation. And I don't think people asked many questions either. People were compliant, very much so. For example, I got a lot of needles at school and never asked what they were for.

In some ways, the hospital was worse than residential school because people were so isolated. There was nowhere to go. I think the feeling of the patients, when I worked there, was of being locked in. It was always a complaint. A lot of people got so impatient with being sick and having to be isolated in the hospital.

I remember visiting Thom Paul, who I knew from back home. He wanted to be out fishing, and he looked so healthy, yet he couldn't go. He was frustrated. I've only heard one person talk about that frustration, and that's my cousin. Now that I think about it, I know in the earlier years the hospital staff were very strict. If you left the hospital or ward you could be arrested because you were spreading disease.

NURSING AIDE AT LAC LA RONGE
NURSING STATION

Muriel Innes

I interviewed Muriel Innes in May 1999 as part of a project that I
was doing about nursing in northern Saskatchewan. We talked in
her backyard in Saskatoon. She was keen to tell me about her work
as a young woman. Her work as a nurses' aide in the Lac La Ronge
Hospital was a way for her father to keep her nearby while the family
earned an income. Muriel lived at the hospital while she worked. She
felt that it gave her a good career for a time.

~~~~~~~~~~~~~~~~~~~~~~~~~~~~

I BECAME A NURSES' AIDE at the nursing station in La
Ronge when I was sixteen. I moved to La Ronge from Bangor,
Saskatchewan, in May 1949 when my father got a job as a foreman
at the fish plant there. My mom had passed away, and my father
thought it would be a good idea for me to work at the hospital. My

half-sister also moved to La Ronge with us, and she worked at the fish plant with Dad. I think I worked at the hospital for two or three years. I was on paid probation at first. That lasted from the summer until the fall of 1949. After that, I was a regular staff member. I recall I wore a uniform with white shoes, and stockings and a pin.

The nursing station—it was really a small hospital—at La Ronge was located on the main floor of the building, and the nurses lived upstairs. There was an extra room in the hospital where people stayed sometimes. I remember the RCMP stayed there once when there was a drug addiction case in town. The nurses at the station were on duty twenty-four hours a day, with only two hours off every second evening. They had to work hard!

My duties were to fold and sterilize gauze, help administer ether during deliveries, administering needles, and making beds. I remember lots of women were encouraged to come to the station to have their babies back then. Just in case something happened. I don't remember any patients ever dying in childbirth. Only one baby died that I remember. It was attributed to SIDS, and no one blamed the hospital. All the nurses I worked with were quite experienced, and we tried to work at keeping our standards high. The nurses were very dedicated to their work, but I don't think they ever really mingled with the community. They had too much work to do.

The nurses were quite interested in attending to women and their babies. They wanted to change how the Indian women cared for their babies. For example, new mothers were encouraged to use cloth diapers instead of the traditional moss bags. I think the mothers went along with this until they left the hospital because they accepted the nurses' strict system, and that was just the way things were done in the hospital. Once they got home, they reverted to their traditional ways.

There were all kinds of diseases and illnesses that came through. Things like fish poisoning, and injuries caused by fishhooks. And I also remember one case of leukemia. There were very few male patients. Most of the patients were women who came in for pregnancy or childbirth.

Once, when one of the nurses broke her leg, I had to step in and take over some of her work. I was sent out to assess and bring patients into the hospital. They did tell me to be careful about who I brought in, though, because some people just wanted a free ride! Sometimes I escorted patients with TB to Prince Albert, where there was a sanatorium. My mom had died of TB, so I was immune. I also helped screen patients for TB during the treaty days. Patients wouldn't get their treaty money until they had taken their medicine. It didn't matter if patients were treaty, non-treaty, or white—we treated everyone.

I also worked in the hospital garden. We stored produce from the garden in the root cellar, and we used that to feed patients with. Our nurses didn't speak Cree, so it was our cook at the hospital who acted as our translator. I had to supervise the cook, the maintenance man, and the cleaner. They were all older than me, but they had to follow my instructions. I also learned to smoke at the hospital.

One of the hardest times at the hospital was during fall freeze-up and spring break-up, when planes couldn't land because conditions weren't safe. This often lasted three to six weeks and was quite hard on the patients because they couldn't be flown out. We also couldn't get any supplies flown in. We had to have all kinds of contingency plans in case of an emergency. The nurses did have all kinds of transportation for travel—float planes and snow planes, like Norsemans and Cessnas, and a Beaver. They also used dog sleds and cutters. Sometimes the Bombardier snow machines. The bush pilots were really fabulous.

After La Ronge, I transferred to the Indian hospital that was in the old army hospital at North Battleford. I did think of leaving there, and I was interested in maybe going to Inuvik, until I met a nurse who worked there. She was so big and strong, I thought maybe I shouldn't go north like that. Instead, I went to Prince Rupert, where there was another Indian hospital. There were lots of Native nurses at those hospitals. I thought of attending nursing school myself, but I couldn't really afford to.

ABORIGINAL PEOPLE AND NURSING

Evelyn Voyageur

During the spring of 2009, I attended a gathering of Elders where I
met Evelyn Voyageur, a retired registered nurse now working as an
Elder-in-Residence at North Island College in the community of Comox
on Vancouver Island. Knowing about her long career, and noting her
commanding presence, I asked Dr. Voyageur if she would be interested in describing her experience becoming—and being a nurse—to
me. I was surprised that she replied with great and unreserved
enthusiasm, "Yes!" A busy woman, it was clear she was still eager to
participate in nurse training and educating anyone who would listen
about cultural issues. She is a regular featured speaker at conferences
and workshops and at the time of writing was vice-president of the
nationally active Aboriginal Nurses Association of Canada.

In reviewing her life's decisions and activities, a relatively clear
relationship emerges between the history of formal health care in
Aboriginal communities and the trajectory of her life. Although
Dr. Voyageur is more than her career, perhaps her story can illustrate

how Canada's approach to Aboriginal health, as well as the connections between health and formal education, affects individuals and their communities. The legacy of the authoritarian approaches shared by Indian Health Services and the Indian Residential Schools system in Canada cannot be ignored much longer.

Dr. Voyageur's life is a testimony to how Aboriginal people have coped with a health care system that, for decades, was not open to influence by their communities in a formal or fundamental manner. Yet, her history also shows that the same system was still affected by the presence of individuals who sought to change it, if even on a personal level.

~~~~~~~~~~~~~~~~~

I COME FROM THE KINGCOME INLET BAND (Tsawataineuk Band) at Kingcome of the Kwakwaka'wakw Nation. I was raised in Kingcome Inlet and at Gilford Island, our neighbouring village, where my grandmother is from, before going to the residential school. I went to the residential school in Alert Bay until grade nine. I was raised by my parents and was very close to my grandmothers. My grandfathers passed on before I knew them, but both my grandmothers, paternal and maternal, were a big part of my life. My dad's mom died when I was seven, but my maternal grandmother lived to see my children. So I was very fortunate to have both my grandmothers and my parents with me when I was small.

The fact that they didn't go to the residential school has a big impact on my life today. Apparently my dad's dad kept my dad out of school because he saw his older son and his nephews returning from this residential school and saw they had no more skills or hope in life from being in the school. This was the school that my parents were forced to put their children in. Because of what he observed, my grandfather said to my dad, "I don't want you to go because those who were there are lost. They don't know how to live; they don't know how to cope in life."

So my dad was hidden when the children were sent off to school. It was good that my dad didn't go. For her part, my mother apparently went for half a day until she saw a relative of hers in Alert Bay village, so she ran away. This relative was an unusual person. She was really for changing the world, and she hid my mother. People thought she supported the school, but she didn't. She took my mom and would never let her go back to the school.

I am very, very lucky that my parents and grandmothers didn't go to such a residential school. In doing my own studies, I have seen what an impact such institutions have had down through many generations. So I grew up, and my parents were very, very cultural. They lived by our culture. In fact, my dad left us lots of tapes of songs and stories. That was our past time when we were young! Singing and telling stories. We were on the go all the time. My parents worked very hard, even though they didn't have what you might now call jobs. When Dad came home after working, he would sing for us. It was really wonderful. I know that my upbringing gave me strength later in life, and when I was sent to school.

I went to the residential school at the age of nine. My parents went to a meeting one day and my mom came back crying. She said I had to go to school, or they would go to jail. That's all I remember of that. To this day, I have tried to remember, how did I get to that school? Did my dad take me on his boat? One of the ladies from our area said we were put on a water taxi, and that there were ten of us. We were sent to Alert Bay that way. I have no recollection of that boat trip, or even of walking up to the school. I have memories of being in the school, but how I got there, I think I blocked that.

I went to residential school and I always say that the school tried to mould us into something else. We lost our identity there because everything was foreign. Although we spoke our language when we arrived, we weren't allowed to speak it at school. We even had to learn to eat stuff we were not familiar with. We had to share our rooms with fifty other kids. I couldn't talk to my brother who was on the other side, and we had to line up for everything—for food, for showers, to go pray. We prayed about four or five times a day to a god we were told would punish us if we were disobedient.

St. Michael's Indian Residential School in Alert Bay was an Anglican school. In my mind, it was less evil than the other residential schools, even though it's not worth comparing these schools. I denied having any issues stemming from my experiences in the school. I was not physically or sexually abused, so I always said, "Oh, I didn't have any problems." Not until I became a nurse did I start feeling like something was wrong, and I confirmed that when I started to further my education. In those days, you stopped school when you were sixteen. There was no encouragement for you to get higher education. The government said we were going to be labourers.

In my time, the policy was that we were not going to be educated, and we were a threat to the non-Native world because we might take away their jobs. So, after school I went home and got married when I was eighteen and a half, and had three children. When I was twenty-five, my husband passed away. This was when the government started allowing us to have further education. I didn't want to sit at home and be a welfare person all my life, so I decided to go back to school. I was in Kingcome, and I started somehow. By correspondence I upgraded my grade nine. And then I moved down to Victoria to finish my grade ten at the vocational school. My cousin took my children and looked after them for me.

While I was in Victoria, I thought, "What do I want to do? What should I do next?" I don't think it was planned at that time that I would be a nurse. They were still not encouraging us to do academics, but because they saw I was doing so well in school—I was really good in math and English and had won $100 from the Department of Indian Affairs because my grades were so good—so they said good for her, and [encouraged] me to become a practical nurse. So I did. The program was right next door to where I did my grade ten. That's where I did my practical nurses' training.

Even at that time there was a lot of racism. I remember the principal of that school complained to me about that. He tried to warn me about how hard it might be for me. He said I had two strikes against me—one was that I had to prove that I could become a nurse, and second that I had to put up with a structured program that was very racist. They were very good teachers in the program, I was told, but they were very racist. He tipped me off. I guess my saving grace was that there was a coloured girl in the nursing program, as well, and they picked on her more often in class. Until she was in tears. She was my friend! They picked on her more, and I bet if she hadn't been there I would've been their number one choice. I won an award there, when I finished. That program was about a year or so. I think I graduated in 1963. Then I went to work in the veteran's hospital in Victoria. That's where I met my second husband. We got married and we moved to Vancouver.

I think at that time I really had the desire to know more about nursing. Maybe I wanted to know more because of the experiences I had when I was a child. When I was small, the nurses came to our villages to treat us and no explanation was given whatsoever to our parents about what they were doing. They would just grab us and poke us. They didn't tell us anything. My mom began to hide us when she knew the nurse was coming. She said, "We don't know what they're putting in you—they don't tell us! For all you know they might be killing us all." So she would begin to hide us. I guess that was on my mind when I went on in my education.

I went for my RN. I attended Langara Community College nursing school, and went there for a year and a half. I didn't fail any exams, except one instructor failed me on the very last thing, which was my bedside nursing. One of the other instructors came to me, and she was very upset about what had happened to me. So I dropped out of there, but I didn't give up. I thought, "I'm not going to let them get me down." I went to Douglas College to challenge the exam—I had seen an ad in the newspaper that practical nurses could challenge the exam to be allowed to continue training to become a registered nurse. Unfortunately, I was very sick on the day of that exam. I had a really bad flu, but I tried to do the exam anyway.

I guess the instructor who was overseeing us writing our exams saw me. She came over and asked me if I was okay. I told her I was sick. I got most of it done, but I was anxious after that to find out how I had done. Later, I called in and asked how I did. It turned out I was one of the top ten out of one hundred! I should always be sick when I write exams!

I will always be grateful for getting into that Douglas College. The teachers were more understanding. They were more inclined to listen to their students. There were quite a few of us practical nurses, and two weeks after we wrote our exam we were all called in to do a refresher course and learn some more. The lady that failed me—going back to her—I met her years later at a conference where I was speaking, and she tried to apologize to me. I also heard later that she treated another Native the same way. I tried to help in that situation. It is important for people to understand how hard it was for us a students, what happened to us. I try to tell people about it now so it can change. Just imagine, that teacher at Langara could've destroyed my life if I hadn't pressed on. It was no secret to the higher-ups in the school as to what she was doing to Native students, but no one did anything about it. So that was my experience in nursing school. I will always be grateful for Douglas College and those special teachers who encouraged, rather than discouraged, me.

I worked in the hospitals as an LPN in North Vancouver, and then as an RN in Langley and later other places. I never had trouble finding work. I got a call from Alberta, and after sending in my résumé and doing an interview, I got a job at Fort Chipewyan. There were no doctors there. It was a federal nursing station—Medical Services branch. It was 1979 when I first went to work there. It was a five-nurse station. This was in the time when there was a drive towards devolution of health care services to Aboriginal communities—we were supposed to close down our federal service and begin making plans so that the community could take over their own health care. But it struck me as strange because at that time the community itself was not making any plans. It was the federal nurses who were doing the planning. That was the start of devolution. It's a treatment centre more, there.

Before I went up there I had to go around with a doctor in the Charles Camsell Indian Hospital to get oriented. It was because of my experiences in northern Alberta that I began to realize there was more to the problems in the villages than simply poor health. There was something more that was causing problems in communities—the problems stemmed from something. It was really surprising to me that people weren't helping themselves. It was my husband who said, "You have to remember, the people in the villages are residential school survivors."

We didn't have positive role models: we didn't see our parents look after our children, there was no caring at the schools. People were treated like an assembly line at those schools. So I began to think, "Yes, there is more to know about this than what they teach us as nurses in university." So I asked, "Are there any programs where I can learn more? I really need to understand where the people are coming from."

So I went to a program at the Nechi Institute, in St. Albert, Alberta—an alcohol- and drug-counselling program for people who want to take it. It was a twenty-five-day course. The first ten days are basic counselling, and the next are advanced. The last five days are all about "you." It was the best thing I'd ever had to do. Until then I really denied having any problems from the residential school, but when I found out more and began dealing with emotions, a lot of it came out. I was always the biggest critic of my family when I saw them drinking. I couldn't understand why they would do that. Now I know that it's the pain they are trying to cope with. This is how they cope with their traumatic experiences. Now I can be more empathetic, rather than critical of them.

There were other nurses who took the course, and there were those nurses who walked out of that because they didn't believe in such a thing. They didn't think it was worthwhile. To this day, I know that experience is a great asset. There is a lot more to our problems in health. I was at Fort Chip for five years, and I know I made a difference because I got a compliment from my nursing supervisor. She said, "You know, I notice that the people are more independent when you are with them. You made a difference in their lives."

When she worked there, the people were constantly at the door at all hours, so I know I made a difference because I showed them that I cared and that I wanted to work *with* them, not work for them or help them. They had to help themselves. There is a big difference. A lot people have trouble understanding that big difference. If nurses come into the villages and say, "I've come to help you," then I say to them, "Get out!" But if they say, "I've come to work *with* you," if they want to work hand in hand with people to find their own solutions, then they are welcome.

In time, I had to leave Fort Chip. My mother was getting quite old and my dad had died, so I needed to come home. I applied for a job at Bella Bella, on the coast. I was there for a short time. I worried about coming back to my people and seeing their problems, the emotional problems that affect their overall health. Then I got a call from a physician at Port Hardy—they needed someone there. I was there for fourteen years.

That was also Medical Services. In the late 1990s, devolution of health care services from the federal government to First Nations continued, but I wasn't ready to work for any of the tribal councils because I saw the unhealthiness of the leaders—they still had the mentality of the Department of Indian Affairs and the residential schools. Even today I see that. So I didn't want to work for them.

I covered seven villages when I was in Port Hardy. I covered three villages from Bella Bella. There was quite a bit of travel involved. When I was working in Port Hardy my goal was getting the villages together. I thought it was important to do what you normally do in our culture—get people together. One of the Elders told me this was important.

When I moved to Port Hardy I made some changes that I thought important—I didn't want to follow the established way of having the nurse follow the doctor around and just "parachute" into communities when there was a problem. You can't establish relationships that way, or build them. So I started staying overnight in the villages and bring in programs. I truly believe that people have to see us as a person, not just as a nurse. They need to know that you are a human being who can relate to them at their level.

I am sorry to say that these changes are now taken away, now that Intertribal Health has taken over. They just come in to drop in a program now and then, and they have started individualizing services. Separating homecare from community health from long-term health, and all those things. Our people didn't understand why there were so many nurses coming and going! They couldn't understand, and those nurses all had different things to say. All these different nurses confused the people—the people didn't like it. I was an all-in-one package. But things have changed—the policies, the legal things.

Nowadays, if you are a community health nurse you can't do a health nurse program. For example, one of the complaints from one of the villages was about how the nurse would come and just sit there. She couldn't go visit. And the people in the village would tell her, "You will be more successful if you go out and visit." Nowadays there is too much liability, and policies create a lot of problems.

I remember one of my supervisors once asking me, "How can you treat your own family?" I consulted an Elder to talk to me about that. As far as I'm concerned, I'm very objective. I treat people the same. I don't have a problem with that. I asked the Elder if I should stop treating my family. And he said, "Evelyn, what did we do before the health system came? If our medicine men or healers were here, they would treat a sick person, no matter who they were. They wouldn't refuse because they were family. It's our tradition. We treat them all the same. Tell them that."

Even after those experiences I still wanted to know more. I had a supervisor who did her master's degree in Seattle. I went to Bastyr University, and they have a very holistic and healthy program. That's where I did my master's program. Other people I knew went there, and they were very happy with that program. It was a very expensive program, but I really wanted to go. It allowed me, again, to deal with many of my own issues that I hadn't dealt with. I realized I still had some issues from my residential school time. It was very helpful. The instructors there were very helpful and tried to help me with what I was experiencing. It allowed me to voice things that I had never shared.

Then I thought, "Well, I need to write all that down," so that's why I went on to do my PHD. I really studied the issues that affect our people. After that I knew I was okay. For my research, I interviewed a lot of people, and some of them were afraid to speak about their experiences, such as residential school—they were afraid their abusers would know who they were. But they wanted to speak because they wanted the younger generations to understand what they went through.

I knew about the Indian hospitals and I knew a lot of our people went there. As I said, we've not dealt with the impact of the hospitals. It should be addressed. Our people that went there were guinea pigs—I'm not sure if you know, but a lot of people today who were in the hospitals, many have only one lung. They did lobectomies on lungs, removed lungs and all those kinds of things. I've heard many stories, even about people who didn't have tuberculosis being put in the Indian hospitals. The hospitals got money from the government for the number of patients they had. The patients were often there for years. And there was a lot of research being done on people. New surgeries and drugs were tried.

These kinds of things were in the back of my mind when I was looking to understand what was happening to our people. Especially when I went to northern Alberta and saw things written in the charts about how people were treated at the Indian hospitals. The Camsell patients were sterilized and there was little consent. I read those things in patient charts. Some of the patients I met were victims of this Indian Hospital system. It was quite disturbing for me. Children would die in the Indian hospitals and they were buried wherever. I know examples of where that happened. It was almost like the parents had no say whatsoever in their children's lives once those children were in the hospital. Sometimes parents never even knew where their children were sent. Not much of this seems to be documented.

In 1999 I retired from nursing. I went to work with the residential school healing program for about four years. We worked to help people talk and begin healing, and to talk about the effects of the schools on our health. That is my passion today.

What I really want to bring forward is cultural awareness and First Nations. There is a real lack of cultural awareness information about First Nations in schools of all kinds and in books. There is nothing about how to work with people from the residential schools. In fact, there is a lot of stereotyping in the books. The information is too general. For example, sometimes they say eye contact is not a part of First Nations traditions. Yet, if my grandmother was speaking to me and I didn't look at her, she would know something was wrong.

When I went to the University of Victoria there was nothing about First Nations. For example, they had a multicultural day, and everybody was there but First Nations. The immigrant ladies were telling their stories, but no First Nations were present. My cousin and I, Maggie Sedgemore, would be very vocal. After a while they started asking us questions. We even did a cultural awareness for the homecare workers in Victoria. We wanted people to understand that homecare was part of health. So we did that. I always laugh because we did all that without pay.

At the university, the professors got the money and got us to do their tasks for them. We were never paid. We felt so strongly about this work that we wrote a letter to the dean, and we met with her to present our ideas for teaching. Fourteen years from the time that we approached her, Maggie and I were called by the University of Victoria, asking us to bring our curriculum ideas forward. I went to the meeting with a group of First Nations nurses, and then they asked us to apply to write up the curriculum. Maggie and I didn't get chosen, even though it was our idea! They chose a Métis woman and a non-Native woman. You'd think they'd choose local women who knew these cultures here. Again, I went to an Elder. I wanted to know what to do. They told me to stay on it, and keep working on it. They told us not to give up. So I did. Everything they wrote we helped with, and it turned out well. Now that material is an elective course for nurses' training.

Then I got another call to help develop cultural competency training. Again, I went to UVic and worked on it. I worked with a social worker from the interior and a community health aide from Tsartlip, and a few others. That course can be used by anybody—it's a program that gets used often.

The curriculum has to change. It has to be more inclusive. We have had opposition from the academic world, but how can they ignore culture? North Island College pioneered change in their own nursing curriculum. We had a chief from Kingcome approach us and suggest that we bring the nursing students to the culture! He said, "Why is it always us having to come to your turf? Try the other way— come and live with us, and learn all about us."

Joanna Fraser, who I work with, she figured it out and she got funding to start a program to do this. So Joanna and I took ten students to the village. The entire community was involved in edu- cating these nurses! We held the classes in our big house, and the nurses lived with families in the village. The nurses saw and felt it all. North Island College is so different—it's become culturally aware, and has pioneered this. We teach the nurses to build rela- tionships—it's a different philosophy. I think this is my life's work. Today I'm working as an Elder-in-Residence at North Island College here in Comox, where I want to teach cultural awareness. It's a good feeling to think how far we've come.[1]

POSTSCRIPT

ABORIGINAL PEOPLE HAVE BECOME ACTIVE in asserting their
own approaches to health care as a response to the legacy of IHS.
Treatment institutions have evolved to support Aboriginal perspectives in health care, such as the Nechi Institute in Alberta, founded
in 1974 as an Aboriginal addictions services centre and training institute.[1] In 1975 the Registered Nurses of Canadian Indian Ancestry
(RNCIA) was launched to support Aboriginal nurses within their profession, followed by the formation of a provincial body, the Manitoba
Indian Nurses Association.[2] Nurse training has also changed to
include more input from Aboriginal peoples, now featuring more
cultural awareness training for non-Aboriginal health care workers.

As IHS devolved its health care responsibilities to local smaller
facilities across Canada, initiatives aimed at employing Aboriginal
people to support community health also gained ground in the 1970s;
by the 1980s more than three thousand community health representatives and health liaison workers worked at the community level.[3] The

story of these community health aides and liaison workers is one that still needs telling. In this way, by the twenty-first century, federal delivery of health services to Indian and Inuit people has moved from a service centred on hospitals and federally controlled administrative units to a more diffuse system based, in theory, on increased community control and provincial involvement in health care provision. More and more, Aboriginal people have begun to reclaim their involvement in health and wellness services, programs and activities.

As late as 1998, however, research dealing with Aboriginal women and formal health care revealed that, in spite of need, "health care services are either not available or not adequately used by Aboriginal women in Canada due to a lack of culturally appropriate care" and prejudice.[4] The recollections of Evelyn Voyageur, featured in this volume, certainly give insight into this claim.

The devolution of health care services from federal to more local Aboriginal control has been uneven and continues to this day. Although Aboriginal peoples are increasingly integrated into Canada's universal public health care system, the impact of Indian Health Services and its facilities and staff remains tangible, continuing to influence the evolution of new services and health care worker training.

ACKNOWLEDGEMENTS

WITHOUT THE GENEROSITY AND PATIENCE of many different people this book could not have been completed. Over the years, many individuals contributed their stories, their suggestions and critical insights, as well as funds and time to my effort of creating a manuscript and then reworking that into book form. It is my hope this final creation honours their individual and collective efforts.

First and foremost, I am grateful to my teachers. Maria Campbell, Florence James, Ray Peter and Florence Elliott, Ellen Rice White, and Delores Louie all shaped my understanding of indigenous stories, storytelling, and the art of bringing human experiences to paper. Not only did they train me to take my time but also to "sit, watch and listen," to hear, and finally to find my own way of expressing stories shared with me. They accompanied me on interviewing visits and encouraged me over several years. Their teachings continue to influence my understanding of life and how to write about it.

I especially want to thank those individuals who shared their stories for trusting me to publish their—often deeply personal—experiences as Aboriginal peoples within a government health care system: Kathleen Steinhauer, Gilbert Anderson, Laura Cranmer, Violet Charlie, Sainty Morris, Evelyn Voyageur, Michael Dick, Marie Dick, Violet Clark, Delores Louie, and Muriel Innes. I am also thankful for the memories of Rae Dong, Truus van Royen, Marjorie Warke, and Mary Crisp. I would not have come to study this topic with the same sense of responsibility had I not encountered and spent time with two significant women—nurses—who worked at the Mt. Edgecumbe Hospital in Sitka, Alaska: Marjorie Ward and Marlys Tedin. They were the first to introduce me to what life in an Indian Health Service hospital was like. I will always be indebted to them.

Authors and scholars who came before me provided many significant examples of how I might understand and work with oral history and life narratives. Pioneering works by Julie Cruikshank, Jo-ann Archibald, Gerald Vizenor, Neal McLeod, Wendy Wickwire, Freda Ahenakew, and George Blondin sit on my bookshelf at home, quietly and unobtrusively serving as sources of inspiration for me.

Colleagues from various universities supported me during my ongoing research into the history of Aboriginal health and Indian Health Services. I acknowledge my colleagues Phyllis Fast, William Schneider, and Walkie Charles of the University of Alaska; my good friends and colleagues Brenda Macdougall at the University of Saskatchewan, Sonya Grypma at Trinity Western University, and Melody Martin at Vancouver Island University. Lesley McBain, at First Nations University of Canada, worked extensively with me on aspects of this book and shared her expertise on the history of northern nurses in Saskatchewan and Alberta. All of these people inspired me in their own way and provided critical feedback on many occasions. Patricia Geddes and Sylvia Scow were very helpful with their assistance regarding transcriptions when I ran into trouble.

Carol Sheehan of cs Communication Strategies deserves special acknowledgement for her editorial talents. She worked tirelessly to help me to polish a rough manuscript into a readable text. Her skill and patience are extraordinary. Without her help the manuscript would not have been finished.

The research presented here was funded in part by the Social Sciences and Humanities Research Council of Canada through their Standard Research Grant program. I derived additional support from my family, especially my mother, who always reminded me of the subject's significance, came on research trips with me, read versions of the manuscript, and would not let me give up. Finally, thank you to Don, who helped me every day on this long journey.

Laurie Meijer Drees
Ladysmith, British Columbia

APPENDICES

APPENDIX 1

IHS Nursing Staff and Field Stations, 1946–1970

All numbers derived from Department of National Health and Welfare, *Annual Reports, Indian Health Services.* Specifically, Canada, House of Commons, Sessional Papers, Department of National Health and Welfare, *Annual Report, Indian Health Services* (1946–47), 32–33; Canada, House of Commons, Sessional Papers, Department of National Health and Welfare, *Annual Report, Indian Health Services* (1961–62), 9.

YEAR	IHS HOSPITALS	NURSING STATIONS (not including health centres or clinics)	NURSING STAFF (field and hospital)
1946–47	18	22	119
1951–52	18	30	275
1961–62	19	43	696
1970	14	64	No record

IHS *Operations and Capital Expenditures, 1950–1963*

All numbers derived from Ottawa, Indian and Northern Affairs, Claims and Historical Research Centre, Indian Affairs Branch, "Health Services for Indians," file L.14, 2.

YEAR	STAFF	OPERATIONS EXPENDITURES	CAPITAL EXPENDITURES
1950–51	1200	$7,859,812	$1,280,031
1954–55	1600	$12,605,043	$935,591
1958–59	1959	$16,403,799	$2,449,187
1962–63	2634	$18,000,000	$1,427,200

NOTES

1. In *Healing Histories: Stories from Canada's Indian Hospitals* I use the terms *Aboriginal* and *indigenous* to refer generally to Canada's First Peoples. The term *First Nations* is used here in reference to Status Indian people as defined by Canada's *Indian Act*. Although Indian Health Services (IHS) was created to provide health care to Status people, Métis and Inuit were also affected by the government service, and so I chose to generalize my terminology. Naturally, all interpretations offered here are my own and any errors should be attributed to me.

2. James B. Waldram, D. Ann Herring, and T. Kue Young, *Aboriginal Health in Canada: Historical, Cultural and Epidemiological Perspectives* (Toronto: University of Toronto Press, 1995), 176, commented on this divergence: "It is clear...that there was no grand strategy for the development of government services for Aboriginal peoples. Such development occurred on an ad hoc basis depending on the region, the legal status of the Aboriginal group in question, and even the personalities of the various caregivers and administrators who, in one way or another, were charged with the responsibility for Aboriginal health."

3. Truth and Reconciliation Commission of Canada, Introduction, accessed April 22, 2011, http://www.trc.ca/websites/trcinstitution/index.php?p=7.

4. Julie Cruikshank, in collaboration with Angela Sidney, Kitty Smith, and Annie Ned, *Life Lived Like a Story: Life Stories of Three Yukon Native Elders* (Vancouver: University of British Columbia Press, 1987);

Julie Cruikshank, *The Social Life of Stories: Narrative and Knowledge in the Yukon Territory* (Vancouver: University of British Columbia Press, 1998), xii–xiii.

5. Neal McLeod, *Cree Narrative Memory: From Treaties to Contemporary Times* (Saskatoon: Purich Publishing Limited, 2007), 8–9. McLeod follows a tradition of Saskatchewan Aboriginal scholars, including Winona Stevenson and Maria Campbell, who are concerned with indigenous narratives and "story." See Winona Stevenson, "Decolonizing Tribal Histories," PHD thesis, University of California Berkeley, 2000; Maria Campbell, *Stories of the Road Allowance People* (Penticton, BC: Theytus Books, 1995). Others, such as Cree scholar Freda Ahenakew, Dene writer George Blondin, Nlha7kapmx scholar Darwin Hanna, and anthropologist Wendy Wickwire, have worked tirelessly to document First Nations' family and community stories in an effort not only to document them but also to bring that narrative history forward to a larger audience, thereby adding to the cultural diversity of historical understanding. See Freda Ahenakew and H.C. Wolfart, eds., *Kohkominawak Otacimowiniwawa: Our Grandmothers' Lives as Told in Their Own Words* (Saskatoon: Fifth House Publishers, 1992); Darwin Hanna and Mamie Henry, eds., *Our Tellings: Interior Salish Stories of the Nlha7kapmx People* (Vancouver: University of British Columbia Press, 1995); Wendy Wickwire, ed., *Living By Stories: A Journey of Landscape and Memory* (Vancouver: Talonbooks, 2005); and George Blondin, *Trail of the Spirit: The Mysteries of Medicine Power Revealed* (Edmonton: NeWest Press, 2006).

6. Jo-ann Archibald, *Indigenous Storywork: Educating the Heart, Mind, Body and Spirit* (Vancouver: University of British Columbia Press, 2008), ix. Her research on Coast Salish peoples taught her that stories, both traditional and personal, are rooted in culturally specific ways of understanding and thus convey to listeners ways of being, thinking, and learning. In her words, "It is important to appreciate the diversity among Indigenous cultures and to recognize that there are different story genres, purposes, protocols and ways to make story meaning." (83) She emphasizes how stories serve as teachers to people, educating the heart, mind, body, and spirit (x, 112–14, 153). My experience working with oral histories related to IHS demonstrated that the powerful stories I collected had the same function.

7. Archibald emphasizes how storywork involves the principles of respect, responsibility, reciprocity, reverence, holism, and interrelatedness. Although I did not have access to her work during my own research, my experience reflects those principles as working methods. Archibald, *Indigenous Storywork*, ix.

Neal McLeod, in his excellent discussion of Cree narrative memory, characterizes the workings of narrative in a similar fashion, indicating that it "is ongoing, and is sustained through relationships, respect and responsibility." McLeod, *Cree Narrative Memory*, 18.

8. Florence James in conversation with Laurie Meijer Drees, Penelakut, British Columbia, April 25, 2011.

9. Shawn Wilson, *Research Is Ceremony: Indigenous Research Methods* (Halifax: Fernwood Publishing, 2008), 79.

10. I was drawn to consider the role of autobiographical statements by the opinions of various authors found in Mark Kramer and Wendy Call, *Telling True Stories: A Non-Fiction Writers' Guide From the Nieman Foundation at Harvard University* (New York: Plume, 2007), 65–83.

11. Mary-Ellen Kelm, *Colonizing Bodies: Aboriginal Health and Healing in British Columbia, 1900–1950* (Vancouver: University of British Columbia Press, 1998). Kelm, who has conducted research into the history of formal Western health care and Aboriginal peoples, suggests a state of medical pluralism existed in First Nations communities in the twentieth century (171–72). By this, she argues that First Nations would use their own remedies and cures when Western medicine appeared to fail them. As I will develop in subsequent chapters, the stories shared with me imply something slightly different—that local or traditional healing practices and notions of health were never really subsumed to Western medicine.

12. Joseph Bruchac, *Our Stories Remember: American Indian History, Culture and Values through Storytelling* (Golden, CO: Fulcrum Publishing, 2003), 35.

INTRODUCTION

1. Mary-Ellen Kelm, *Colonizing Bodies: Aboriginal Health and Healing in British Columbia 1900–1950* (Vancouver: University of British Columbia Press, 1998), 122.

2. Canada, Indian Health Services and Indian Affairs Branch, *Circular Letter to All Superintendents, Indian Agency, Regional Supervisors, and the Indian Commissioner for BC, and to all Medical Officers, Indian Health Services*, File L.3 (Ottawa: Claims and Historical Research Centre, 1953).

3. Ibid.

4. For additional information on the Indian Residential Schools system in Canada see J.R. Miller, *Shingwauk's Vision: A History of Native Residential Schools* (Toronto: University of Toronto Press, 1996); John S. Milloy, *"A National Crime": The Canadian Government and the Residential School System—1879 to 1986* (Winnipeg: University of Manitoba Press, 1999); E.M. Furniss, *Victims of Benevolence: Discipline and Death at the Williams Lake Indian Residential School, 1891–1920* (Williams Lake, BC: Cariboo

Tribal Council, 1992); Madeleine Dion Stout and Gregory D. Kipling, *Aboriginal People, Resilience and the Residential School Legacy* (Ottawa: Aboriginal Healing Foundation, 2003).

5. Kelm, *Colonizing Bodies*, 129, 151–52. Kelm argues that medical pluralism existed in British Columbia's Aboriginal communities, and that this practice functioned as a form of resistance to the colonizing intention of Indian Health Services. I hope to build on her insight by featuring actual descriptions of the work of indigenous "medicine" by patients themselves.

Laura Cranmer

1. "Cold Needles" is an unpublished play by Laura Cranmer. Excerpt printed with permission.

1

TUBERCULOSIS

1. Ethel Martens, "Culture and Communications: Training Indians and Eskimos as Community Health Workers," *Canadian Journal of Public Health* 57, no. 11 (November 1966): 495.
2. Stefan Grzybowski and Edward A. Allen. "Tuberculosis: 2. History of the disease in Canada," *Canadian Medical Association Journal* (April 6 1999): 1025–28.
3. R.M. Jasmer, P. Nahid, and P.C. Hopewell, "Clinical Practice. Latent Tuberculosis Infection," *New England Journal of Medicine* 347, no. 23 (2002): 1860–66.
4. World Health Organization, "Tuberculosis," Fact Sheet 104 (2007).
5. N.E. Flanders, "Tuberculosis in Western Alaska, 1900–1950," *Polar Record* 23, no. 145 (1987): 383–96, 384.
6. Mark Caldwell, *The Last Crusade: The War on Consumption, 1862–1954* (New York: Athaneum, 1988), 16–39.
7. Thomas Dormandy, *The White Death: A History of Tuberculosis* (New York: New York University Press, 2000), 105–25.
8. Ibid, 262–63. See also Katherine McCuaig, *The Weariness, the Fever and the Fret: The Campaign Against Tuberculosis in Canada, 1900–1950* (Montreal and Kingston: McGill-Queen's University Press, 1999), 93, 99.
9. McCuaig, *The Weariness*, 29–30.
10. Ibid.
11. Grzybowski and Allen, "Tuberculosis," 1026.
12. Janice P. Dickin McGinnis, "The White Plague in Calgary: Sanatorium Care in Southern Alberta," *Alberta History* 28, no. 4 (Autumn 1980): 1–15.

13. Laurie Meijer Drees, "Reserve Hospitals and Medical Officers," *Prairie Forum* 21, no. 2 (1996): 149–76.

14. Caldwell, *The Last Crusade*, 247.

15. Georgina D. Feldberg, *Disease and Class: Tuberculosis and the Shaping of Modern North American Society* (New Brunswick, NJ: Rutgers University Press, 1995), 2–3.

16. McCuaig, *The Weariness*, 85.

17. Pat Sandiford Grygier, *A Long Way from Home: The Tuberculosis Epidemic Among the Inuit* (Montreal and Kingston: McGill-Queen's University Press, 1994), 3–5.

18. McCuaig, *The Weariness*, 211, 218, 269.

19. Caldwell, *The Last Crusade*, 266–68.

20. Liz Ruskin, "Drug combinations slowed TB spread," *Anchorage Daily News*, July 30, 2000, A10.

21. Caldwell, *The Last Crusade*, 270. See also Elfrida Nord, "The War on Tuberculosis in Alaska, 1945–1960: A Look at the Role of Public Health Nursing," *Alaska History* 9, no. 2 (1994): 45–51.

22. Bruce Noton, "Northern Manitoba Treaty Party, 1949," *Manitoba History* 39 (Spring/Summer 2000): 1.

23. Statistics are derived from Matt Mattas, "What is Tuberculosis?" in *The Camsell Mosaic: The Charles Camsell Hospital, 1945–1985*, edited by Charles Camsell History Committee (Altona, MB: Charles Camsell History Committee, 1985), 249. These statistics are supported by those offered in G. Graham-Cumming, "Health of the original Canadians, 1867–1967," *Medical Services Journal of Canada* 23, no. 2 (1967): 134. Graham-Cumming indicates that rates of tuberculosis in the Indian population were five times the Canadian average in 1967. He further points out how, based on a Dominion Bureau of Statistics report on tuberculosis among Indians and Inuit between 1950 and 1952, active tuberculosis was estimated to be 12.3 times the national rate (138).

24. G.J. Wherrett. *The Miracle of the Empty Beds: A History of Tuberculosis in Canada* (Toronto: University of Toronto Press, 1997).

25. Feldberg, *Disease and Class*, 163–64.

2

INDIAN HEALTH SERVICES

1. Ottawa, Indian and Northern Affairs Canada, Claims and Historical Research Centre, file L.14, "Canada's Indian Health Services," speech delivered in the radio series, *Report from Parliament Hill*, Paul Martin, Minister of National Health and Welfare, March 29, 1947.

2. Canada, *House of Commons Debates* (6 June 1952), p. 2987 (Paul Martin, Minister of National Health and Welfare).
3. Kathleen Steinhauer, interview with Laurie Meijer Drees, Edmonton, Alberta, August 25, 2004.
4. Canada, House of Commons, Sessional Papers, Department of Indian Affairs, *Annual Report* (1930), 93.
5. See Canada, House of Commons, Sessional Papers, Department of Indian Affairs, *Annual Report* 14 (1896), 8–12; *Annual Report* 27 (1905), 165–66; *Annual Report* (1929), 11.
6. James B. Waldram, D. Ann Herring, and T. Kue Young, *Aboriginal Health in Canada: Historical, Cultural and Epidemiological Perspectives* (Toronto: University of Toronto Press, 1995), 163.
7. T. Kue Young, *Health Care and Cultural Change: The Indian Experience in the Central Subarctic* (Toronto: University of Toronto Press, 1988), 90–91.
8. P.G. Nixon, "Percy Elmer Moore (1899–1987)," Arctic Profiles, *Arctic* 42, no. 2 (June 1989): 166–67.
9. Ibid, 166–67.
10. G. Graham-Cumming, "Health of the Original Canadians, 1867–1967," *Medical Services Journal of Canada* 23, no. 2 (1967): 123. He points out how governmental services for Indian health grew "under pressure of growing need and public outcry..."
11. Provincial Archives of Alberta, Accession No. 96.2/7, file 1, "Indian Health Services," speech, 1949, 4.
12. Canada, House of Commons, Sessional Papers, Department of National Health and Welfare, *Annual Report, Indian Health Services* (1946–1947), 32. See also Ron Bergmann, "Trials and Tribulations," in *The Camsell Mosaic: The Charles Camsell Hospital, 1945–1985*, edited by Charles Camsell History Committee (Altona, MB: Charles Camsell History Committee, 1985), 45.
13. G.J. Wherrett, "Survey of Health Conditions and Medical and Hospital Services in the North West Territories (Part I, Arctic Survey)," *The Canadian Journal of Economics and Political Science* 11 no. 1 (February 1945): 54–55.
14. Mary Crisp, interview with Laurie Meijer Drees, Comox, British Columbia, July 8, 2010.
15. Canada, House of Commons, Sessional Papers, Department of National Health and Welfare, *Annual Report, Indian Health Services* (1949–50), 80.
16. Canada, House of Commons, Sessional Papers, Department of National Health and Welfare, *Annual Report, Indian Health Services* (1947–48), 41.
17. Canada, House of Commons, Sessional Papers, Department of National Health and Welfare, *Indian and Northern Health Services* 16, no. 2, supplement no. 38 (1961).
18. Canada, House of Commons, Sessional Papers, Department of National Health and Welfare, *Annual Report, Indian Health Services* (1951–52), 49.

19. Canada, House of Commons, Sessional Papers, Department of National Health and Welfare, *Annual Report, Indian Health Services* (1949–50), 82.

20. Ibid, 50.

21. For example, the Blackfoot Indian Hospital in Gleichen, Alberta, was originally established as a mission hospital by the Church of England in the 1890s, but it was rebuilt into a larger modern facility in the 1920s. This unusual expansion was made possible through the use of band funds held in trust by the Department of Indian Affairs. In the 1940s, this facility operated forty beds under the auspices of IHS. The larger Charles Camsell Indian Hospital, in comparison, was a refurbished American military hospital, as were several of the smaller northern hospitals.

22. Canada, House of Commons, Sessional Papers, Department of National Health and Welfare, *Annual Report, Indian Health Services* (1948–49), 107. See also Canada, Department of National Health and Welfare, *Indian and Northern Health Services* 16, no. 2, supplement no. 38 (1961).

23. Canada, House of Commons, Sessional Papers, Department of National Health and Welfare, *Annual Report, Indian Health Services* (1953–54), 42.

24. Canada, House of Commons, Sessional Papers, Department of National Health and Welfare, *Annual Report, Indian Health Services* (1948–49), 107.

25. As noted by P.G. Nixon, Moore continued in his public service role until his retirement in 1965. From 1956–59 he was chairman of the World Health Organization, and after his retirement he remained an active member of the Canadian Lung and Canadian Tuberculosis Associations.

26. See Canada, House of Commons, Sessional Papers, Department of National Health and Welfare, *Annual Report, Indian Health Services* (1945); and *Annual Report, Medical Services* (1971).

27. Ethel Martens, "Culture and Communications: Training Indians and Eskimos as Community Health Workers," *Canadian Journal of Public Health* 57, no. 11 (November 1966): 495.

28. Canada, House of Commons, Sessional Papers, Department of National Health and Welfare, *Annual Report* (1960), 435.

29. Young, *Health Care and Cultural Change*, 91.

30. Waldram, Herring, and Young, *Aboriginal Health in Canada*, 165.

31. Health and Welfare Canada, "The Transfer of Health Services to Indian Control," *Saskatchewan Indian Federated College Journal* 4, no. 1 (1988): 8.

32. Waldram, Herring and Young, *Aboriginal Health in Canada*, 179–81.

33. Ibid, 179, 180.

34. The idea of "moral imagination" is developed by American intellectual historian Gertrude Himmelfarb in her book, *Poverty and Compassion: The Moral Imagination of the Late Victorians* (New York: Alfred A. Knopf, 1991).

Elva Taylor

1. The complete interview, including the comments and questions of the interviewer, is held on tape in the Provincial Archives of Alberta's Charles Camsell Hospital Interview Collection (Tape 92.129/6). See also Annalisa R. Staples and Ruth L. McConnell, *Soapstone and Seed Beads: Arts and Crafts at the Charles Camsell Indian Hospital, A Tuberculosis Sanatorium* (Edmonton: The Provincial Museum of Alberta, 1993).

3

THE INSTITUTIONS

1. Canada, *House of Commons Debates* (21 June 1951), p. 4450; and *House of Commons Debates* (6 June 1952), p. 2987.
2. Canada, House of Commons, Sessional Papers, Department of National Health and Welfare, *Annual Report, Indian Health Services* (1951–52), 49.
3. C. Richard Maundrell, "Indian Health: 1867–1940," unpublished MA thesis, Queen's University, 1941, 10, 15, 39. "A questionnaire sent in 1933 to the Agents in the Territories showed that the evidence of non-pulmonary tuberculosis was very high evidence of low resistance...the epidemic is much severer today in the north," 39.
4. Canada, House of Commons, Sessional Papers, Department of National Health and Welfare, *Annual Report, Indian Health Services* (1947–48), 41.
5. Canada, House of Commons, Sessional Papers, Department of National Health and Welfare, *Annual Report* (1967), 73.
6. Canada, House of Commons, Sessional Papers, Department of National Health and Welfare, *Annual Report, Indian Health Services* (1946–47), 32.
7. Michael Dick, interview with Laurie Meijer Drees, June 2, 2008, Nanaimo, British Columbia.
8. Delores Louie, interview with Laurie Meijer Drees, May 27, 2008, Cedar, British Columbia; Violet Charlie, interview with Laurie Meijer Drees, May 14, 2008, Duncan, British Columbia.
9. Violet Clark, interview with Laurie Meijer Drees, July 3, 2008, Nanaimo, British Columbia.
10. Charles Camsell History Committee, eds., *The Camsell Mosaic: The Charles Camsell Hospital, 1945–1985* (Altona, MB: Charles Camsell History Committee, 1985), 43, 95, 98.

11. Canada, House of Commons, Sessional Papers, Department of National Health and Welfare, *Annual Report, Indian Health Services* (1945–46), 26.

12. W. Lynn Falconer, "Historical Record—Charles Camsell Hospital," in Charles Camsell History Committee, eds., *The Camsell Mosaic*, 5.

13. Canada, *House of Commons Debates* (1948 Volume VI) p. 5322 (Paul Martin, MP).

14. Charles Camsell History Committee, eds., *The Camsell Mosaic*, 249.

15. Ibid, 98.

16. Herbert Roberts, "The Camsell Buildings and Their Problems," in Charles Camsell History Committee, eds., *The Camsell Mosaic*, 9.

17. Ibid, 8.

18. In 1958, the Camsell Hospital became partially accountable to the Alberta provincial Department of Health under the new universal health care program in Canada, which was administered by the provinces. The impact on the Camsell was that it had to change its accounting practices to verify the costs of care of Indians in hospital for anything other than tuberculosis care.

19. Canada, House of Commons, Sessional Papers, Department of National Health and Welfare, *Annual Report, Indian Health Services* (1948–49), 108.

20. Canada, House of Commons, Sessional Papers, Department of National Health and Welfare, *Annual Report, Indian Health Services* (1950–51), 65.

21. Canada, House of Commons, Sessional Papers, Department of National Health and Welfare, *Annual Report, Indian Health Services* (1951–52), 49.

22. Provincial Archives of Alberta, Accession No. 96.2/7, file 1, *Financial Post*, 6 January 1961.

23. Canada, House of Commons, Sessional Papers, Department of National Health and Welfare, *Annual Report, Indian Health Services* (1951–52), 49.

24. National Archives of Canada, Northern Affairs Program, 1947, RG 85, C-1-a, Vol. 1015, file 17877, Mrs. Muriel Schonbert, RN, *Report Prepared for the National Film Board of Canada*, 3.

25. Canada, House of Commons, Sessional Papers, Department of National Health and Welfare, *Annual Report, Indian Health Services* (1952–52), 34.

26. Provincial Archives of Alberta, Accession No. 92.48, Box GSE, no file, G.C. Gray, *Stepping Stones to Health: Information for T.B. Patients* (Edmonton: Charles Camsell Indian Hospital, 1962). Also, patient comments in *Lost Songs*, directed by Clint Tourangeau, National Film Board of Canada, 2000, videocassette.

27. Gray, *Stepping Stones to Health*.

28. Ibid.

29. An excellent overview of the diagnosis and treatment of tuberculosis in Canada is featured in Pat Grygier's work, *A Long Way From Home: The Tuberculosis Epidemic Among the Inuit* (Montreal and Kingston: McGill-Queen's University Press, 1994), 3–15.

4

PATIENTS AND FAMILIES

1. Simon Saimaiyuk and Sarah Saimaiyuk, "Life as a TB Patient in the South," *Inuktitut* 71 (1990): 24.
2. Kathleen Steinhauer, interview by Laurie Meijer Drees, Edmonton, Alberta, August 25, 2004.
3. Annalisa R. Staples and Ruth L. McConnell, *Soapstone and Seed Beads: Arts and Crafts at the Charles Camsell Indian Hospital, A Tuberculosis Sanatorium* (Edmonton: The Provincial Museum of Alberta, 1993), 12.
4. Saimaiyuk and Saimaiyuk, "Life as a TB Patient in the South," 20, 23.
5. See interviews featured here, the *Camsell Arrow* accounts, as well as recollections published in Charles Camsell History Committee, eds., *The Camsell Mosaic: The Charles Camsell Hospital, 1945–1985* (Altona, MB: Charles Camsell History Committee, 1985).
6. Beatrice Calliou, "I was one of the first patients at the Charles Camsell Hospital," in Charles Camsell History Committee, eds., *The Camsell Mosaic*, 96.
7. Gilbert Anderson, interview with Laurie Meijer Drees, Edmonton, Alberta, August 25, 2004.
8. Staples and McConnell, *Soapstone and Seed Beads*, 13–25.
9. Ibid, 2, 27–28.
10. Ibid, 12.
11. W.L. Falconer, regional superintendent, Indian and Northern Health Services, 1961, quoted in Ibid, 9.
12. The *Camsell Arrow* is reproduced and held on microfilm at the Provincial Archives of Alberta. Editions of the *Camsell Arrow* used here derived from Accession No. 69.73 (Roll 1, May 1947 to August 1951; Roll 5, October 1955 to October 1956; Roll 7, Spring 1962 to Christmas 1965) and Accession No. 67.73 (Roll 2, August 1951 to April 1954). Fred Dew, principal, writing in the *Camsell Arrow*, March/April 1952, 13.
13. Kathleen Steinhauer, interview by Laurie Meijer Drees, Edmonton, Alberta, August 25, 2004.
14. Ellen White, interview by Laurie Meijer Drees, Nanaimo, British Columbia, April 10, 2005.
15. Doreen Callihoo, "It Just Isn't the Same Anymore," in Charles Camsell History Committee, eds., *The Camsell Mosaic*, 99.

16. Provincial Archives of Alberta, *Camsell Arrow* microfilm, Accession No. 69.73, Roll 1, Dr. M. Matas, *Camsell Arrow*, 23 May 1947, 1.
17. *Camsell Arrow*, 8 July 1947.
18. *Camsell Arrow*, 23 May 1947.
19. *Camsell Arrow*, March/April 1950, 4.
20. *Camsell Arrow*, January/February 1956, 1.
21. *Camsell Arrow*, March/April 1950, 11.
22. *Camsell Arrow*, March/April 1956, 71.
23. Ibid, 72.
24. *Camsell Arrow*, May/June 1952, 11–12.
25. *Camsell Arrow*, Autumn 1962, 66.
26. *Camsell Arrow*, March/April 1950, 11.
27. Staples and McConnell, *Soapstone and Seed Beads*, 11.
28. Ottawa, Indian and Northern Affairs Canada, Claims and Historical Research Centre, file L.14, p. 2, "Indian Rehabilitation and Integration Services that are being promoted by the Indian Affairs Branch, Department of Citizenship and Immigration," presentation at the Annual Meeting of the Canadian Tuberculosis Association at Niagara Falls, 16 May 1956.
29. Fred Dew, "The Rehabilitation Program," in Charles Camsell History Committee, eds., *The Camsell Mosaic*, 196.
30. Ibid. In 1961 the Edmonton rehabilitation program was discontinued.
31. Ottawa, Indian and Northern Affairs Canada, "Indian Rehabilitation and Integration Services," 6.
32. *Camsell Arrow*, March/April 1956, 27–28.
33. Violet Clark, interview by Laurie Meijer Drees, Nanaimo, British Columbia, July 3, 2008.
34. Sainty Morris, interview by Laurie Meijer Drees, Nanaimo, British Columbia, November 30, 2007.
35. Michael Dick, interview by Laurie Meijer Drees, Nanaimo, British Columbia, June 2, 2008

Alma Desjarlais

1. Provincial Archives of Alberta, Charles Camsell Hospital Interview Collection, Tape 92.129/18.

5

1. A version of this chapter has been published as a research note in *Histoire sociale/Social history*, Volume 43, Number 85, May 2010, 165–191.
2. Mary-Ellen Kelm, *Colonizing Bodies: Aboriginal Health and Healing in British Columbia, 1900–1950*. (Vancouver: University of British Columbia Press, 1998), 127–29.
3. Kathryn McPherson, "Nursing and Colonization: The Work of Indian Health Service Nurses in Manitoba, 1945–1970," in *Women, Health, and Nation: Canada and the United States Since 1945*, edited by Georgina Feldberg, Molly Ladd-Taylor, Alison Li, and Kathryn McPherson (Montreal and Kingston: McGill-Queen's University Press, 2003) 223–46; 232–34.
4. Kelm, *Colonizing Bodies*, 153; McPherson, "Nursing and Colonization," 234.
5. McPherson, "Nursing and Colonization," 235.
6. My interviews took place in 2005 and 2009.
7. Kelm, *Colonizing Bodies*, 164.
8. This discussion of *snuwuyulth* is based on information shared with me by Florence James (Penelakut First Nation), Ray Peter (Cowichan Tribes), Delores Louie (Chemainus First Nation), and Ellen White (Snuneymuxw First Nation) between 1999 and 2009 as part of my work in the First Nations Studies Department, Vancouver Island University. Descriptions of such teachings are missing from the standard ethnographies dealing with Coast Salish cultures, including Homer G. Barnett, *The Coast Salish of British Columbia* (Eugene, OR: University of Oregon, 1955); Wayne Suttles, *Coast Salish Essays* (Vancouver: Talonbooks, 1987). Luckily, an excellent source for understanding Coast Salish worldviews has been released: Bruce Granville Miller, ed., *Be of Good Mind: Essays on the Coast Salish* (Vancouver: University of British Columbia Press, 2007).
9. Ethnobotanist Nancy J. Turner has written extensively on plant use on British Columbia's coast. Examples of her older works include: Nancy J. Turner, John Thomas, Barry F. Carlson, and Robert T. Ogilvie, *Ethnobotany of the Nitinaht Indians of Vancouver Island*, British Columbia Provincial Museum Occasional Papers Series No. 24 (Victoria: The British Columbia Provincial Museum and Parks Canada, 1983); Nancy J. Turner, Laurence C. Thompson, M. Terry Thompson, Annie Z. York, *Thompson Ethnobotany: Knowledge and Usage of Plants by the Thompson Indians of British Columbia*, Royal British Columbia Museum, Memoir No. 3 (Victoria: Royal British Columbia Museum, 1990). More recent works feature plant and resource use more broadly: Douglas Deur and Nancy J. Turner, eds. *Keeping it Living: Traditions of Plant Use and Cultivation*

on the *Northwest Coast of North America* (Vancouver: University of British
Columbia Press, 2005).

10. Ellen White, interview with Laurie Meijer Drees, Nanaimo, British
Columbia, October 25, 2007.

11. Delores Louie, interview with Laurie Meijer Drees, Cedar, British
Columbia, May 28, 2008.

12. Violet Charlie, interview with Laurie Meijer Drees, Duncan, British
Columbia, May 14, 2008.

13. Kelm also mentions the importation of grease into the Indian hospital
setting in her work on Indian Health Services before 1950, *Colonizing
Bodies*, 163–64.

14. Accessed May 16, 2008, http://www.wellsphere.com/
healthy-eating-article/oolichan-grease-and-my-big-fat-diet/548833.

15. Accessed May 16, 2009, http://www.cbc.ca/thelens/bigfatdiet/grease.
html; and accessed May 16, 2009, http://www.livinglandscapes.bc.ca/
northwest/oolichan_history/preserving.htm.

16. Wolfgang G. Jilek, *Salish Indian Mental Health and Culture Change* (Toronto:
Holt, Rinehart and Winston of Canada, 1974), 105.

17. Personal communication with Florence James, Nanaimo, British
Columbia, May 2010.

18. Historian Kathryn McPherson has shown that it is important to research
and theorize the diverse, and often oppositional, ways women relate to
their health care systems, by extension, it is important to research and
theorize how cultural minorities relate to those same standard systems
in society. See McPherson, "Nursing and Colonization," 241.

6

WORKING IN HEALTH CARE

1. A version of this chapter has been published as a paper in the *Canadian
Bulletin of Medical History* 27, no. 1 (2010): 139–62.

2. Provincial Archives of Alberta, Charles Camsell Hospital Fonds, PR 0383,
1946–1988, PR 1991. p. 93, Dr. W.L. Falconer, Assistant Superintendent of
Medical Services, to the Director, Indian Affairs Branch, Ottawa, 10 June
1942.

3. G.J. Wherrett, "Survey of Health Conditions and Medical and Hospital
Services in the North West Territories (Part I, Arctic Survey)," *The
Canadian Journal of Economics and Political Science* 11, no. 1 (February 1945):
57.

4. National Archives Canada (NAC), RG 29, Vol. 2934, file 851-1-x300, pt. 2,
Medical Services Branch, Saskatchewan Region, J. Kirkbride to Dr. B.F.
Habbick, Prince Albert, Saskatchewan, 12 April 1973.

5. Kathleen Steinhauer, interview by Laurie Meijer Drees, Edmonton, Alberta, August 25, 2004.

6. J. Rick Ponting and Roger Gibbins, *Out of Irrelevance: A Socio-political Introduction to Indian Affairs in Canada* (Toronto: Butterworths, 1980), 140.

7. See T. Kue Young, *Health Care and Cultural Change: the Indian Experience in the Central Subarctic* (Toronto: University of Toronto Press, 1988), chapters one and two. Northwestern Canada or "western subarctic" includes the region west of Hudson Bay, including the northern Prairie provinces, the Northwest Territories, and Yukon. Young refers to the western subarctic as a region that has no precise boundaries but includes lands south of the Arctic tundra treeline, and coincides with the boreal forest and zone of discontinuous permafrost of the central and western provinces to the northern territories and Alaska (9). IHS was most active in this region as provincial institutions took over the care of indigenous patients in southern areas. IHS focused its attention on serving indigenous populations in areas where no provincial services were available—generally, the middle and far North.

8. Michael Dick, interview with Laurie Meijer Drees, Nanaimo, British Columbia, June 2, 2008. Also confirmed by Kathleen Steinhauer, interview by Laurie Meijer Drees, Edmonton, Alberta, August 25, 2005.

9. Yukon Archives, Whitehorse, RG 85, C-1-a, Vol. 791, file 6210, Dr. Ross Miller, Director of Medical Services, Department of Pensions and National Health to R.A. Gibson, Deputy Commissioner, Northwest Territories Branch, Department of Mines and Resources, 28 November 1939.

10. Yukon Archives, Whitehorse, RG 85, C-1-a, Vol. 791, file 6210, Extract from Bishop Turquetil's letter to Mr. R.A. Gibson, Deputy Commissioner, Northwest Territories Branch, 19 February 1940.

11. Yukon Archives, Whitehorse, RG 85, C-1-a, Vol. 791, file 6210, Extract from the *Minutes of the One Hundred and Thirty Second Session of the Northwest Territories Council*, 2 October 1941, 3.

12. Yukon Archives, Whitehorse, RG 85, C-1-a, Vol. 791, file 6210, *Proceedings of the Committee Authorized by Minutes of the Northwest Territories Council Meeting of 9 October 1941 to Consider the Training of Indian Girls in the Hospitals of the Northwest Territories*, 3.

13. G.J. Wherrett, who was responsible for surveying health conditions in the Arctic in 1945, made a brief mention of the program and the need to cooperate with the schools. See G.J. Wherrett, "Survey of Health Conditions," 57.

14. Ibid, 55.

15. Yukon Archives, Whitehorse, RG 85, C-1-a, Vol. 791, file 6210, probably Dr. J.A. Urquhart to R.A. Gibson, Director, Lands, Parks and Forests Branch, Department of Mines and Resources, 27 February 1940.

16. Yukon Archives, Whitehorse, RG 85, C-1-a, Vol. 791, file 6210, *Proceedings of the Committee Authorized by Minutes of the Northwest Territories Council Meeting of 9 October 1941 to Consider the Training of Indian Girls in the Hospitals of the Northwest Territories*, 1.

17. Yukon Archives, Whitehorse, RG 85, C-1-a, Vol. 791, file 6210, Extracts from the *Minutes of the One Hundred and Thirty-Second Session of the Northwest Territories Council*, 20 October 1941, Dr. Moore on record.

18. Yukon Archives, Whitehorse, RG 85, C-1-a, Vol. 791, file 6210, Dr. J.A. Urquhart to R.A. Gibson, Director, Lands, Parks and Forests Branch, Department of Mines and Resources, 8 December 1941. The members of this group of "graduates" had clearly already been in some sort of training program devised by the Fort Smith mission hospital and were awarded their "certificate" as soon as the document was given government endorsement. The example stands to reveal that Aboriginal "nurse" training occurred in an informal manner in remote locations before government-sponsored initiatives became prominent.

19. Wherrett, "Survey of Health Conditions," 55.

20. Muriel Innes, interview by Laurie Meijer Drees and Lesley McBain, Saskatoon, Saskatchewan, May 1, 1999.

21. Ottawa, Indian and Northern Health Services, Directorate Report, 1960, 13.

22. Ottawa, Indian and Northern Health Services, Directorate Report, 1960, 13.

23. Canada, *House of Commons Debates* (6 June 1952), p. 2988. The Hon. Paul Martin was Minister for the Department of National Health and Welfare from 1946–1957, and as such was responsible for IHS.

24. Percy E. Moore, "Health for Indians and Eskimos," *Canadian Geographical Journal* 48, no. 6 (June 1954): 216–21. Photograph appears on p. 220 of the journal.

25. Charles Camsell History Committee, eds., *The Camsell Mosaic: The Charles Camsell Hospital, 1945–1985* (Altona, MB: Charles Camsell History Committee, 1985), 162.

26. Ottawa, Indian and Northern Health Services, Directorate Report, 1960, 44.

27. Ibid.

28. Charles Camsell History Committee, eds., *The Camsell Mosaic*, 196–97.

29. Ottawa, Indian and Northern Health Services, Directorate Report, 1961, 9.

30. Ottawa, Indian and Northern Health Services, Directorate Report, 1960, 41.

31. Ottawa, Indian and Northern Health Services, Directorate Report, 1959, 213.

32. Ottawa, Indian and Northern Health Services, Directorate Report, 1960, 41.

33. Wilma Major quoted in Kathryn McPherson, *Bedside Matters: The Transformation of Canadian Nursing, 1900–1999* (Don Mills, ON: Oxford University Press, 1996), 213.

34. Indian and Inuit Nurses of Canada, "Special Awards," *Newsletter* 1, no. 1: 2–3.

35. Ibid, 3–4.

36. See "Indian Women," *Saskatchewan Indian* (March 1989): 12; "Celebrating Women's Achievements, Canadian Women in Science, Jean Cuthand Goodwill, Nurse," accessed May 26, 2003, http://www.nlc-bnc.ca/2/12/h12-406-e.html.

37. Kathleen Steinhauer, interview by Laurie Meijer Drees, Edmonton, Alberta, August 25, 2004.

38. Ibid.

39. Ibid.

40. Violet Clark, interview by Laurie Meijer Drees, Nanaimo, British Columbia, July 3, 2008.

41. Jean Cuthand Goodwill, "Indian and Inuit Nurses of Canada," *Saskatchewan Indian* (March 1989): 14–18. Other First Nations women went even further abroad than the United States. Martha Soonias, originally of the Red Pheasant Reserve, attended a mothercraft course in Toronto before leaving for New Zealand, where she qualified as a registered midwife. She returned to Canada to assume a nursing position at the new Battleford Indian Hospital in 1948. See "Statement of MP Mr. Bater, June 21, 1951," in Canada, *House of Commons Debates* (21 June 1951), p. 4453.

42. Canadian Nurses' Association quoted in McPherson, *Bedside Matters*, 211.

43. Ibid, 205, 209, 210–11.

44. Ellen White, interview by Laurie Meijer Drees, Nanaimo, British Columbia, October 25, 2007.

45. Library and Archives of Canada, RG 29, Vol. 2982, file 851-5-x300, pt. 1, K.A. Mellish, "A Report on the Environmental Sanitation Conferences of the Indian and Northern Health Services Directorate, Saskatchewan Region."

46. Ibid, 9, 12.

47. Ottawa, Indian and Northern Health Services, Directorate Report, 1961, 9.

48. Paul Roach, "Sanitation Workshop for Indians," in *Canada's Health and Welfare* (May 1960): 3.

49. Mary Jane McCallum, "The Early History of Community Health Representatives," unpublished paper, May 2006, 4.

50. Alice K. Smith, "Indian and Eskimo health auxiliaries," in *Circumpolar Health, Proceedings of the 3rd International Symposium*, edited by Roy J. Shephard and S. Itoh (Toronto: University of Toronto Press, 1974), 591–92.

51. Ethel G. Martens, "Culture and Communications: Training Indians and Eskimos as Community Health Workers," *Canadian Journal of Public Health* 57, no. 11 (November 1966): 495.

52. Ibid, 497.

53. Ibid, 502.

54. Dr. Percy Moore, "The Modern Medicine Man," in *People of Light and Dark*, ed. Maja van Steensel (Ottawa: Department of Indian Affairs and Northern Development, 1966), 134.

55. McCallum, "The Early History of Community Health Representatives," 8–9. And, Waldram, Herring, and Young argue that CHR program "smacked of tokenism." James B. Waldram, Ann Herring, and T. Kue Young, *Aboriginal Health in Canada: Historical, Cultural and Epidemiological Perspectives* (Toronto: University of Toronto Press, 2000), 253.

56. Martens, "Culture and Communications," 502.

57. Ibid.

58. Ottawa, National Archives of Canada, RG 29, Vol. 3053, Interim Box 41, file 853-1-1, pt. 2, Memorandum, Director General, Medical Services, 2 December 1969.

59. Ottawa, Indian and Northern Affairs Canada, Claims and Historical Research Centre, Medical Services overview, February 1978, p. 23, Table 13.

Evelyn Voyageur

1. Personal communication with Evelyn Voyageur, Comox, British Columbia, April 10, 2009.

POSTSCRIPT

1. Information on the Nechi Institute accessed May 6, 2009, http://www. nechi.com/discover/history.php.

2. Jean Cuthand Goodwill, "Indian and Inuit Nurses of Canada," *Saskatchewan Indian Federated College Journal* 4, no. 1 (1988): 95–96.

3. James B. Waldram, Ann Herring, and T. Kue Young, *Aboriginal Health in Canada: Historical, Cultural and Epidemiological Perspectives* (Toronto: University of Toronto Press, 2000), 180.

4. B. Leipert and L. Reutter, "Women's Health and Community Health Nursing Practice in Geographically Isolated Settings: A Canadian Perspective," *Health Care for Women International* 19 (1998): 580.

SELECT BIBLIOGRAPHY

I have included here only a selection of writings and interviews that have
been of direct use or especially influential in the writing of this book. This
bibliography does not represent a complete record of the sources I have
consulted during the research of this project, but might give insight into
how I completed my research. The works may also be of interest to others
wanting more information in this subject area. For further bibliographic
data, please consult the Notes section beginning on page 213.

INTERVIEWS

Anderson, Gilbert. 2004. Interview by Laurie Meijer Drees. August 25.
    Edmonton, Alberta.
Charlie, Violet. 2008. Interview by Laurie Meijer Drees and Delores Louie.
    Tape recording. May 14. Duncan, British Columbia.
Clark, Violet. 2008. Interview by Laurie Meijer Drees. Tape recording. July 3.
    Nanaimo, British Columbia.
Cranmer, Laura. 2008. Interview by Laurie Meijer Drees. Tape recording.
    January 24. Nanaimo, British Columbia.
Dick, Marie. 2008. Interview by Laurie Meijer Drees. Tape recording. June 2.
    Nanaimo, British Columbia.
Dick, Michael. 2008. Interview by Laurie Meijer Drees. Tape recording. June 2.
    Nanaimo, British Columbia.
Dong, Rae. 2010. Communication with Laurie Meijer Drees. April. Ladysmith,
    British Columbia.

Innes, Muriel. 1999. Interview by Laurie Meijer Drees and Lesley McBain.
    May 1. Saskatoon, Saskatchewan.
James, Florence. 2010. Communication with Laurie Meijer Drees. E-mail. May.
    Nanaimo, British Columbia.
Louie, Delores. Interview by Laurie Meijer Drees. Tape recording. May 28.
    Cedar, British Columbia.
Morris, Sainty. 2007. Interview by Laurie Meijer Drees. November 30.
    Brentwood Bay, British Columbia.
Steinhauer, Kathleen. 2004. Interview by Laurie Meijer Drees. Tape recording.
    August 25. Edmonton, Alberta.
van Royen, Truus. 2010. Communication with Laurie Meijer Drees. April.
    Ladysmith, British Columbia.
Warke, Marjorie. 2010. Interview by Laurie Meijer Drees with Carol Sheehan.
    July 2. Comox, British Columbia.
Voyageur, Evelyn. 2009. Interview by Laurie Meijer Drees. Tape recording.
    April 10. Comox, British Columbia.
White, Ellen. 2005. Interview by Laurie Meijer Drees. Tape recording. April 10.
    Nanaimo, British Columbia.
White, Ellen. 2007. Interview by Laurie Meijer Drees. Tape recording.
    October 25. Nanaimo, British Columbia.

GOVERNMENT DOCUMENTS

Canada. *House of Commons Debates.* 1952–70.
Canada. House of Commons, Sessional Papers. Department of Indian Affairs.
    Annual Reports. 1896–45.
Canada. House of Commons, Sessional Papers. Department of National
    Health and Welfare, Indian Health Services. *Annual Reports.* 1946–62.

ARCHIVAL COLLECTIONS

Edmonton Public Library (EPL), Edmonton
    Charles Camsell Hospital Annual *Pictorial Review.*

Glenbow Archives (GA), Calgary
    Joy Duncan's Frontier Nursing Project fonds.

Indian and Northern Affairs Canada, Claims and Historical Research Centre
    (INAC), Ottawa
    Medical Services branch papers.

Library and Archives Canada (LAC), Ottawa
Record Group 85—Northern Affairs.
Record Group 29—National Health and Welfare.

Provincial Archives of Alberta (PAA), Edmonton
Charles Camsell Hospital fonds, 1946–88.
Charles Camsell Hospital Annual *Pictorial Review*.
Camsell Arrow Records, 1947–65.
Joe Atkinson fonds.
Charles Camsell Hospital Interview Collection.

VIDEOS

Tourangeau, Clint. *Lost Songs*. VHS. National Film Board of Canada. 2000.

BOOKS AND ARTICLES

Aboriginal Nurses Association of Canada. *Twice as Good: A History of Aboriginal Nurses*. Ottawa: Aboriginal Nurses Association of Canada, 2007.
Ahenakew, Freda, and H.C. Wolfart, eds. *Kohkominawak Otacimowiniwawa: Our Grandmothers' Lives as Told in Their Own Words*. Saskatoon: Fifth House Publishers, 1992.
Archibald, Jo-ann. *Indigenous Storywork: Educating the Heart, Mind, Body and Spirit*. Vancouver: University of British Columbia Press, 2008.
Barnett, Homer G. *The Coast Salish of British Columbia*. Eugene: University of Oregon, 1955.
Blondin, George. *Trail of the Spirit: The Mysteries of Medicine Power Revealed*. Edmonton: NeWest Press, 2006.
Caldwell, Mark. *The Last Crusade: The War on Consumption, 1862–1954*. New York: Athaneum, 1988.
Campbell, Maria. *Stories of the Road Allowance People*. Penticton, BC: Theytus Books, 1995.
Charles Camsell History Committee, *The Camsell Mosaic: The Charles Camsell Hospital, 1945–1985*. Altona, MB: Charles Camsell History Committee, 1985.
Cruikshank, Julie. *Life Lived Like a Story: Life Stories of Three Yukon Native Elders*. Vancouver: University of British Columbia Press 1987.
———. *The Social Life of Stories: Narrative and Knowledge in the Yukon Territory*. Vancouver: University of British Columbia Press, 1998.

Dickin McGinnis, Janice P. "The White Plague in Calgary: Sanatorium Care in Southern Alberta." *Alberta History* 28, no. 4 (Autumn 1980): 1–15.

Dormandy, Thomas. *The White Death: A History of Tuberculosis*. New York: New York University Press, 2000.

Feldberg, Georgina D. *Disease and Class: Tuberculosis and the Shaping of Modern North American Society*. New Brunswick, NJ: Rutgers University Press, 1995.

Flanders, N.E. "Tuberculosis in Western Alaska, 1900–1950." *Polar Record* 23, no. 145 (1987): 383–96.

Goodwill, Jean Cuthand. "Indian and Inuit Nurses of Canada." *Saskatchewan Indian* (March 1989): 14–18.

————. "Indian and Inuit Nurses of Canada." *Saskatchewan Indian Federated College Journal* 4, no. 1 (1988): 95–96.

Graham-Cumming, G. "Health of the Original Canadians, 1867–1967." *Medical Services Journal of Canada* 23, no. 2 (1967): 115–66.

Grygier, Pat Sandiford. *A Long Way from Home: The Tuberculosis Epidemic among the Inuit*. Montreal and Kingston: McGill-Queen's University Press, 1994.

Halfe, Louise Bernice. *Bear Bones & Feathers*. Regina: Coteau Books, 1994.

Kulig, Judith, and Sonya Grypma. "Honouring Pioneer Aboriginal Nurses from the Blood Reserve." *Alberta RN* 62, no. 8 (2006): 14–16.

Grzybowski, Stefan, and Edward A. Allen. "Tuberculosis: 2. History of the disease in Canada." *Canadian Medical Association Journal* (April 6, 1999): 1025–28.

Hanna, Darwin, and Mamie Henry, eds. *Our Tellings: Interior Salish Stories of the Nlha7kapmx People*. Vancouver: University of British Columbia Press, 1995.

Health and Welfare Canada. "The Transfer of Health Services to Indian Control." *Saskatchewan Indian Federated College Journal* 4, no. 1 (1988): 7–11.

Himmelfarb, Gertrude. *Poverty and Compassion: The Moral Imagination of the Late Victorians*. New York: Alfred A. Knopf, 1991.

Indian and Inuit Nurses of Canada. "Special Awards." *Newsletter* 1, no. 1: 2–3.

"Indian Women." *Saskatchewan Indian*, March 1989.

Jasmer, R.M., P. Nahid, and P.C. Hopewell. "Clinical Practice. Latent Tuberculosis Infection." *New England Journal of Medicine* 347, no. 23: 1860–66.

Jilek, Wolfgang G. *Salish Indian Mental Health and Culture Change*. Toronto: Holt, Rinehart and Winston of Canada, 1974.

Kramer, Mark, and Wendy Call. *Telling True Stories: A Non-Fiction Writers' Guide from the Nieman Foundation at Harvard University*. New York: Plume, 2007.

Kelm, Mary-Ellen. *Colonizing Bodies: Aboriginal Health and Healing in British Columbia, 1900–1950*. Vancouver: University of British Columbia Press, 1998.

King, Thomas. *The Truth about Stories: A Native Narrative*. Toronto: House of Anansi Press, 2003.

Leipert, B., and L. Reutter. "Women's Health and Community Health Nursing Practice in Geographically Isolated Settings: A Canadian Perspective." *Health Care for Women International* 19 (1998): 580.

Martens, Ethel. "Culture and Communications—Training Indians and Eskimos as Community Health Workers." *Canadian Journal of Public Health* 57, no. 11 (November 1966): 495.

Maundrell, C. Richard. "Indian Health: 1867–1940." MA thesis. Queen's University, 1941.

McCallum, Mary Jane. "The Early History of Community Health Representatives." Unpublished paper, 2006.

McCuaig, Katherine. *The Weariness, the Fever and the Fret: The Campaign against Tuberculosis in Canada, 1900–1950*. Montreal and Kingston: McGill-Queen's University Press, 1999.

McLeod, Neal. *Cree Narrative Memory: From Treaties to Contemporary Times*. Saskatoon: Purich Publishing Limited, 2007.

McPherson, Kathryn. "Nursing and Colonization: The Work of Indian Health Service Nurses in Manitoba, 1945–1970." In *Women, Health, and Nation: Canada and the United States Since 1945*, edited by Georgina Feldberg, Molly Ladd-Taylor, Alison Li, and Kathryn McPherson. Montreal and Kingston: McGill-Queen's University Press, 2003.

————. *Bedside Matters: The Transformation of Canadian Nursing, 1900–1999*. Don Mills, ON: Oxford University Press, 1996.

Meijer Drees, Laurie, and Lesley McBain. "Nursing and Native Peoples in Northern Saskatchewan, 1930s–1950s." *Canadian Bulletin of Medical History* 18, no. 1 (2001): 43–66.

Meijer Drees, Laurie. "Reserve Hospitals and Medical Officers." *Prairie Forum* 21, no. 2 (1996): 149–76.

————. "Indian Hospitals and Aboriginal Nurses: Canada and Alaska." *Canadian Bulletin of Medical History* 27, no. 1 (2010): 139–62.

————. "Training Aboriginal Nurses: The Indian Health Services in Northwestern Canada, 1939–75." In *Caregiving on the Periphery: Historical Perspectives on Nursing and Midwifery in Canada*, edited by Myra Rutherdale, 181–209. Montreal and Kingston: McGill-Queen's University Press, 2010.

Miller, Bruce Granville, ed. *Be of Good Mind: Essays on the Coast Salish*. Vancouver: University of British Columbia Press, 2007.

Moore, Percy E. "Health for Indians and Eskimos." *Canadian Geographical Journal* 48, no. 6 (June 1954): 216–21.

Nixon, P.G. "Percy Elmer Moore (1899–1987)." *Arctic* 42, no. 2 (June 1989): 166–67.

Nord, Elfrida. "The War on Tuberculosis in Alaska, 1945–1960: A Look at the Role of Public Health Nursing." *Alaska History* 9, no. 2 (1994): 45–51.

Noton, Bruce. "Northern Manitoba Treaty Party, 1949." *Manitoba History* 39 (Spring/Summer 2000): 15–24.

Ponting, J.Rick, and Roger Gibbins. *Out of Irrelevance: A Socio-political Introduction to Indian Affairs in Canada.* Toronto: Butterworths, 1980.

Roach, Paul. "Sanitation Workshop for Indians." *Canada's Health and Welfare* (May 1960): 3.

Ruskin, Liz. "Drug combinations slowed TB spread." *Anchorage Daily News.* July 30, 2000. A10.

Silko, Leslie Marmon. *Storyteller.* New York: Arcade Publishing, 1981.

Saimaiyuk, Simon, and Sarah Saimaiyuk. "Life as a TB Patient in the South." *Inuktitut* 71 (1990): 24.

Smith, Alice K., "Indian and Eskimo health auxiliaries." In *Circumpolar Health, Proceedings of the 3rd International Symposium,* edited by Roy J. Shephard and S. Itoh, 591–92. Toronto: University of Toronto Press, 1974.

Staples, Annalisa R., and Ruth L. McConnell. *Soapstone and Seed Beads: Arts and Crafts at the Charles Camsell Indian Hospital, A Tuberculosis Sanatorium.* Edmonton: The Provincial Museum of Alberta, 1993.

Stevenson, Winona. "Decolonizing Tribal Histories." PHD diss. University of California, Berkeley, 2000.

Suttles, Wayne. *Coast Salish Essays.* Vancouver: Talonbooks, 1987.

Wickwire, Wendy, ed. *Living By Stories: A Journey of Landscape and Memory.* Vancouver: Talonbooks, 2005.

Waldram, James B., D. Ann Herring, and T. Kue Young, *Aboriginal Health in Canada: Historical, Cultural and Epidemiological Perspectives.* Toronto: University of Toronto Press, 1995.

Wherrett, G.J. *The Miracle of the Empty Beds: A History of Tuberculosis in Canada.* Toronto: University of Toronto Press, 1997.

———. "Survey of Health Conditions and Medical and Hospital Services in the North West Territories (Part I, Arctic Survey)." *The Canadian Journal of Economics and Political Science* 11, no. 1 (February 1945): 54–55.

Wilson, Shawn. *Research Is Ceremony: Indigenous Research Methods.* Halifax: Fernwood Publishing, 2008.

World Health Organization. "Tuberculosis." *Fact Sheet 104* (2007).

Young, T. Kue. *Health Care and Cultural Change: The Indian Experience in the Central Subarctic.* Toronto: University of Toronto Press, 1988.

INDEX

Nanaimo Regional General Hospital
(NRGH), 181, 182
Native Health Worker program, 163
Nechi Institute, 199–200, 205
Nelson, (S. Morris's uncle), XXXII
Noel, Mr. (Camsell staff), 38
North Battleford Hospital, 192
Northwest Territories initiative for
training Aboriginals, 148–51
Norway House Indian Hospital, 45,
163
nurses/nursing
and Aboriginal medicine, 120, 127
Aboriginal women who became,
151–53, 157–61, 169–75, 181
B. Worsley experience of, 29–32
and *Camsell Arrow*, 88–89
at Coqualeetza Indian Hospital,
112–13
and cultural competence,
203–04, 205, 206
E. Taylor's experience as, 34–40
E. Voyageur's experience as, 193,
196–204
Faith's experience as, XLIV–XLV
K. Steinhauer's story of, 169–75
at Lac La Ronge Hospital, 190,
191–92
Michael Dick's experience as, 181
M. Thompson's experience as,
26–28
M. Warke's experience as, 61–67
at Nanaimo Indian Hospital, 102,
117, 119
and public health, 52–56
racism faced by, 160–61, 196–97,
198
trained in US, 157–58
trained overseas, 228n41
T. Van Royen's experience as,
69–72
See also Aboriginals in health care
nursing stations, 24

O'Brien, Miss (Camsell nurse), 89
occupational therapy programs, 83
Ohsweken Reserve, 163
Okpik, Abraham, 38
Onespot, Buddy, 89
oolichan oil (grease), 129–30, 134

Pangnirtung, 31–32
PAS (para-aminosalicylic acid), 8–9,
178
Paul, Thom, 189
Peter, Ray, XX, XXII
physical punishment, XXVIII–XXVIX,
XLV, 112–13, 177
Porter, Ruth, 158
Port Hardy, BC, 200–01
public health
as goal of IHS, 19, 52–56
under Intertribal Health, 201
training Aboriginals in, 162–65,
172, 173, 205
and tuberculosis, 6, 54

racism
at Charles Camsell, 175
in Duncan, BC, 187
in modern health care, 206
at Nanaimo Indian Hospital, 180,
182
and nurses, 160–61, 196–97, 198
in public health, 165
Rapley, Mrs. (Camsell matron), 174
Ray (Elder-in-Residence), XXVI, XXVII
Registered Nurses of Canadian
Indian Ancestry (RNCIA), 205
rehabilitation programs, 94–96, 108
religious services, 109
reserves, 162–65
residential schools
and cultural isolation, 195–96
D. Louie and, 115
effect on survivors, 199
E. Voyageur's time in, 194–96, 202

healing program for, 203
and nursing training, 149
P. Weir's time in, 100
S. Morris's time in, xxvix–xxx,
xxxi–xxxii
St. Michael's, 177–78, 182
tie to IHS, xxxvi–xxxvii, 96–98,
184–85
and tuberculosis, 9
Resolution Indian Residential
School, 149
Rice, Granny, 137, 141
Roberts, Herbert, 51
Roy (L. Cranmer's uncle), 102
Ruby (Nanaimo worker), 185

Sabourin, Gabriel, 90, 92
Saimaiyuk, Sara, 81
Saimaiyuk, Simon, 77
Saskatchewan, 44
Schmidt, Dr. (Nanaimo), 127, 141
Schonbert, Muriel, 54
Sedgemore, Maggie, 203
self-governance of health care.
See devolution of health care
Siksika First Nation, 6
snuwuyulth, 125–26
soapstone carving, 39
Soonias, Martha, 228n41
St. Albert Cemetary, 171, 175
St. Ann's Hospital, 153
Staples, Lisa, 33, 104–10
Steinhauer, Kathleen
on being a doctor, 144
on Camsell, 11, 77, 87, 160
help to author, xx
her story, 168, 169–75
Steinhauer, Ralph, 170
sterilization, 202
St. Michael's Residential School, 100,
177–78, 182, 194–96, 202
storytelling, xviii–xxv, 125, 126–27,
141, 195

streptomycin, 7, 8, 178
Stryker frame, 5, 60
Swindlehurst, Mrs. (Camsell
nurse), 92

Tailfeathers, Rosie, 173
Tallow, Jennie, 173
Taylor, Elva, 33–40, 169–70, 174
Taylor, F.E., 88–89
Thompson, Marge, 26–28
traditional medicine. See Aboriginal
medicine
Truth and Reconciliation
Commission of Canada, xix
tuberculosis
and Aboriginal medicine, xxxiii
Aboriginal rates of, 9, 19, 217n23
in Aklavik, 30
at Charles Camsell, 36, 40, 48, 71,
174–75
drug treatments for, 7–9
history of, 1–6
at Lac La Ronge Hospital, 192
Michael Dick's description of, 177,
178–79
and public health, 6, 54
removal of patients south for
treatment, 16–18
and sanatoria, 6–7, 9, 16
S. Morris's description of, xxviii,
xxxii, xxxiii
surveys, 56, 179
symptoms, xxxv, 1
transmission of, 2–3
treatment at Nanaimo Indian
Hospital, 126, 187–88
treatment regime for, 9–10,
56–60
vaccination for, 7, 10, 14, 197
V. Charlie's experience of, 135–36
V. Clark's experience of, 184, 188
as vehicle for training Aboriginals,
94–96, 154

Tucktoo, David, 90
Turner, Nancy, 125

United States, 157–58
University of Victoria, 203–04
Urquhart, J.A., 150

vaccination, 7, 10, 14, 71, 197
Van Royen, Truus, 68–72
Voyageur, Evelyn, 193–204

Waksman, Selman, 7
Warke, Marjorie, 61–67
Weir, Pearl, 100
Western medicine, XXXVII–XXXVIII,
    130–32
Wherrett, G.J., 16, 143
White, Ellen
    defies hospital rules, 87
    story of, 126–27, 137–42, 161
    on storytelling, XXI, XXII, XXIII
Wilson, Shawn, XXIII
winter spirit ceremonial, 131
Worsley, Biddy, 29–32

Young, T. Kue, 23

OTHER TITLES FROM THE UNIVERSITY OF ALBERTA PRESS

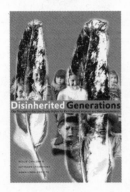

DISINHERITED GENERATIONS
*Our Struggle to Reclaim Treaty Rights for First Nations
Women and their Descendants*
Nellie Carlson & Kathleen Steinhauer,
as told to Linda Goyette
Maria Campbell, Foreword
180 pages • 20 B&W photographs, notes,
appendices, index
978-0-88864-642-2 | $24.95 (T) PAPER
978-0-88864-690-3 | $19.99 (T) EPUB
978-0-88864-691-0 | $19.99 (T) AMAZON KINDLE
Native Studies/Human Rights/Women's Studies/
Oral History

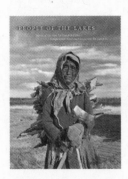

PEOPLE OF THE LAKES
*Stories of Our Van Tat Gwich'in Elders/Googwandak
Nakhwach'ànjòo Van Tat Gwich'in*
Vuntut Gwitchin First Nation & Shirleen Smith
456 pages • Full-colour throughout, 125 colour images
and B&W images, maps, notes, glossary,
bibliography, index
978-0-88864-505-0 | $34.95 (T) PAPER
Native Studies/Oral History/The North

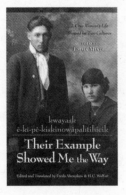

**THEIR EXAMPLE SHOWED ME THE WAY /
KWAYASK E-KI-PE-KISKINOWAPAHTIHICIK**
A Cree Woman's Life Shaped by Two Cultures
Emma Minde
Freda Ahenakew, Translator
H. C. Wolfart, Translator
320 pages • Cree-English glossary
978-0-88864-291-2 | $24.95 (T) PAPER
Biography/Oral History